INTERMITTENT FASTING
FOR WOMEN

Eat Delicious Recipes and Learn with Little Secrets without Effort to Lose Weight Quickly. Improve Your Body and Your Physical Well-Being by Eating with Taste through the Process of Metabolic Autophagy

EMILY ROSS

TABLE OF CONTENTS

INTRODUCTION

I want to thank you for choosing this book, *Intermittent Fasting for Women*, and hope you find the book informative.

The concept of fasting is not a new one and has been around since the dawn of human civilization. However, it has gained popularity only recently because of all the benefits it offers. Intermittent fasting is a brilliant dieting protocol that can help attain your weight loss and fitness goals.

Unlike a lot of other diets, intermittent fasting focuses on *when* you eat instead of *what* you eat. By making certain adjustments to your daily lifestyle, you can reap all the benefits this diet offers. It is quite flexible and can be easily customized. There are several methods of intermittent fasting, and you can choose one according to your needs and requirements.

In this book, you will learn everything you must know about intermittent fasting. You will learn about the basic concepts of intermittent fasting, the benefits it offers, the different protocols of intermittent fasting, and the ways to get started with the diet. Moreover, there are practical tips and strategies in this book that you can follow to keep up your motivation and speed up your weight loss. You will also be given a food list to help you make conscious food choices without breaking your fast. Apart from all this, you will be given plenty of simple recipes to help cook nutritious and delicious meals. All these recipes are quite easy to prepare and will help achieve your weight loss and fitness goals.

So if you are ready, then let us get started without further ado!

CHAPTER 1: INTRODUCTION TO INTERMITTENT FASTING

History of Fasting

The concept of fasting isn't a new one, and it dates back to the dawn of civilization. Fasting has been used throughout human history for different purposes, ranging from medical to spiritual. Fasting is practiced even today and has become rather popular.

What is the first thought that pops into your head when you hear the word "fasting"? You might think about starvation. It is a misconception that fasting and starvation are synonymous. Well, they are nothing alike, and unless you change your mindset about fasting, you will not be able to follow this diet. Starvation isn't voluntarily and is caused by the absence of food. Since it is not deliberate, it cannot be controlled. In starvation, a person doesn't know when they will be able to get their next meal. Fasting, on the other hand, is voluntary. If you voluntarily abstain from consuming any food for whatever the reason, it is fasting. Fasting is not unnatural; it is a common part of life. However, when you abstain yourself from consuming food for specific periods, it is referred to as intermittent fasting.

Fasting is a practice that is common to almost all cultures and traditions across the globe. The father of modern medicine, Hippocrates, believed that fasting frequently is good for one's health. To quote Hippocrates, "To eat when you are sick is to feed your illness." Aristotle, Plato, and other famous thinkers supported the idea of frequent fasts. Ancient Greeks believed that a person's cognitive ability could be improved by fasting. They might have been on to something. How do you feel after stuffing yourself with food or after bingeing on some extremely heavy foods? Do you feel energetic, or do you feel lethargic?

When you stuff yourself with a lot of food, you often feel sluggish, tired, and even sleepy. Whenever you consume a lot of food, your body redirects most of its blood supply to the digestive system. Your body does this to help with better digestion of food. It, in turn, means that the blood supply to your brain decreases. Technically, you are inducing yourself into a state of food coma. Yes, food coma is quite real. All the lethargy that you feel after a heavy meal is because of a shift in your body's metabolism and functioning.

Fasting is a common practice across different religions. Religious scripture shows that Jesus Christ, Buddha, and even Prophet Muhammad believed that fasting had healing powers. In spiritual terms, fasting is believed to have the ability to purify and cleanse one's soul. Not only is fasting an essential part of several religions, but it is also considered to be necessary. Fasting is believed to be beneficial for one's body, mind, and spirit.

During the holy month of Ramadan, Muslims tend to fast from sunrise to sunset. Islamic scripture also supports the idea of fasting twice a week, especially on Mondays and Thursdays. Buddhist monks tend to fast rather frequently. In Jainism, it is a common practice to fast for about a month for religious and spiritual purposes. All religions prescribe fasting as a means of atonement for one's sins.

The idea of fasting has undoubtedly withstood the test of time. Initially, a lot of people believed that fasting was harmful, and they were skeptical about its helpfulness. If it is a dangerous process, don't you think humans would have figured it out by now? Well, fasting cannot harm your body. You will learn more about the different benefits of fasting in the subsequent chapters.

What Is Intermittent Fasting?

Intermittent fasting is not a recent trend. However, this diet started to gain popularity only recently. This simple dieting protocol has taken the world of health and fitness by a storm. Before you learn about the basics of intermittent fasting, you must understand the difference between the two states of our bodies. The first one is the fasted state, and the second one is the fed state. Your body is always in either of these states. The fasted and fed states are two sides of the same coin. If you eat or keep snacking, your body is in a fed state.

In this state, your body is actively engaged in three processes—digestion, absorption, and assimilation. Your body is trying to make the most of the food you eat in this state and stores some energy as reserves for later. Given our modern diets and lifestyles, most of us tend to stay in this state except while sleeping. Now, let us talk about the fasted state. As the name suggests, a fasted state is one wherein your body is fasting. In this state, your body concentrates on burning all the fat stored within to provide energy. All the benefits that intermittent fasting offers are because of your body's transition from fed to a fasted state.

Intermittent fasting is a diet that alternates between periods of eating and fasting. A lot of diets tend to come along with a bunch of dietary restrictions. However, this isn't the case with intermittent fasting.

There are no dietary restrictions, per se. The primary focus of intermittent fasting is not on *what* you eat but *when* you eat. There are different forms of intermittent fasting. Did your fast almost daily? Well, take a moment and think about it. What state do you think your body is in when you are fast asleep? You might not have given it a conscious thought, but you are fasting. Intermittent fasting is merely an extension of this fast your body is in. If you are used to skipping breakfast and eating your first meal at noon, you are effectively fasting. You are essentially fasting for 14–16 hours while the eating window is restricted to about 8–10 hours. Did you know that this is one of the famous protocols of intermittent fasting? Yes, intermittent fasting is as simple as that. Once you get used to fasting, it will come naturally to you. Intermittent fasting encourages your body to stay in a fasted state for as long as possible to speed up the process of burning fats.

Throughout history, humans have fasted for different reasons, ranging from necessity or scarcity of food to even spiritual reasons. Fasting is prescribed by different religions like Christianity, Buddhism, Hinduism, Islam, and even Jainism. In these religions, fasting is used as a means of obtaining spiritual enlightenment. Animals, as well as humans, tend to fast during illness as. The concept of fasting is not unnatural. The human body has been designed in such a manner that it can sustain itself without food for prolonged periods. While you are fasting, different processes tend to change within your body. One of the most straightforward cellular changes that take place in your body is regarding the level of insulin. While fasting, the level of blood sugar in your body decreases, which in turn reduces the need for insulin. This change is especially desirable if your normal blood sugar levels are rather high. You will learn about the different health benefits of intermittent fasting in the subsequent chapters.

Are you wondering what intermittent fasting is about? Once you start following any of the protocols of intermittent fasting, you will be required to fast anywhere between 12 and 48 hours. The eating window, along with the duration of the fast, will depend on the method you choose. When it comes to intermittent fasting, there are no specific rules about what you can and cannot eat. As long as the food choices you make are healthy and you stick to the fasting schedule, it's fine.

Our cavemen ancestors were hunters and gatherers. They could only eat when they found something to eat, so it was quite natural that they used to fast until their next meal. Then along came agriculture and cultivation. Humans no longer had to hunt or work hard to get the next meal. Then came along the industrial revolution that revolutionized the entire food industry. Mass production of food started. The markets are constantly flooded with plenty of food products. The concept of famine slowly started to fade away. Humans are no longer primarily dependent on external environmental factors to obtain food. We no longer have to hunt or gather our food because it is readily available these days. The world has progressed, but biological evolution is still a work in progress. Progress is believed to be not only good but also desirable. It has certainly changed the way we lead our lives these days. However, it is also the reason for the different health problems that humanity faces these days.

How Intermittent Fasting Works

While you are fasting, you are giving your body a recess. Your body gets a chance to cleanse itself internally. When your body is in a fasted state, it no longer depends on the food you consume to provide energy. Instead, it reaches into the stores of fat and starts burning them to provide energy. The genetic makeup of the human body enables us to go on for prolonged periods without consuming any food. The human body is designed such that fasting does not harm it. You might not be aware of it, but our body has plenty of internal resources of fat cells. These reserves are only utilized when you don't consume any food. If you keep consuming food, your body never gets a chance to use these reserves.

Are you aware of the Chinese concepts of yin and yang? This philosophy is based on the idea of dualism. It mainly describes that forces that seem to be opposite might be interdependent, interconnected, and even complementary nature. Yin and yang are two sides of the same coin. It is all about balance. One of the primary laws of nature is the need for balance. This holds true theoretically and practically. If you want your body to function optimally, it needs to have some sort of internal balance. When you apply the concept of balance your body, it essentially means there needs to be a harmony between the fasted and fed states. Your body needs some time to use the stored energy before you can start eating again. Fasting is a recess that your body desperately needs.

Whenever you eat something, your body digests it to provide energy. All the energy that is produced isn't used immediately. A portion of this is stored within for later use. The energy produced from the food you eat is used in two forms. A part of this food is readily converted into glucose, which is used up immediately. The unused glucose is stored in the form of fat cells. Your body saves all the fat in the liver, but the liver has a ceiling limit on the storage space available. Once all the space has been used up, your body starts storing the extra glucose in the form of fatty cells. Your body has plenty of space to store all the fat. In fact, your body will never run out of space to store fat. However, your body doesn't use all the stored energy. If you keep eating, your body will only burn the food you are eating to produce energy but will not access its reserves. If your body has to choose between glucose and fats to provide energy, it will invariably choose glucose. So if you keep eating, you are essentially increasing the reserves of fatty cells. Over a period, this causes weight gain.

Whenever you fast, this process is essentially reversed. When you don't consume any food, you are forcing your body to start using its internal reserves of fat for providing energy. This internal process keeps going on until your next meal. If you provide your body with a constant supply of glucose, it will never get around to burning those fats. So, if you're interested in restoring your body's internal equilibrium, fasting is a good idea. By opting for intermittent fasting, you can help your body restore its balance.

Intermittent fasting is a wonderful dieting protocol, and it can help improve the quality of your life. However, not everyone must opt for this protocol. Any woman who is trying to conceive, pregnant, or breastfeeding must not attempt any form of fasting regardless of its duration. If you have recently undergone major surgery and are recovering from it, fasting is not ideal. If you have to prepare yourself to undergo major surgery or are recovering from any illness, don't attempt fasting. If you have a history of eating disorders or are recovering from one, stay away from fasting.

Fasting can effectively lead to a relapse of an eating disorder. Until you fully recovered, don't attempt fasting. Also, fasting isn't ideal for children. As long as you are healthy adult, intermittent fasting will do you no harm. It might sound as exciting to get started with the new diet, but consult your doctor or healthcare provider before starting intermittent fasting.

CHAPTER 2: BENEFITS OF INTERMITTENT FASTING

Intermittent Fasting on Cellular Level

Whenever you fast, different changes take place in your body. Think of your body as a machine. When you regularly use a machine, its parts undergo significant wear and tear. So once in a while, the machine has to be serviced. Likewise, all the cells in your body also experience inevitable wear and tear due to daily use. So your body also needs maintenance as well as service. At times, cells tend to get damaged, and they need to be either replaced or repaired. When you fast, you are giving your body a break to undertake any repair work. Fasting helps speed up the process of cellular repair. Any damaged cells are either quickly replaced or repaired. Only when your body gets rid of all the damaged cells can it replace them. Intermittent fasting helps in the removal of any toxic waste building up within. Essentially, it helps your body detoxify itself from within. This process is referred to as *autophagy*. You will learn more about autophagy in the subsequent chapters.

Intermittent fasting helps deal with diabetes. Diabetes is a condition wherein the blood sugar levels of an individual are significantly high. Whenever you eat, your body releases insulin to break down the glucose levels building up in your blood. So when you don't eat, your body doesn't have to produce any insulin. By doing this, you can effectively reverse the effects of diabetes on the body. When you are fasting, your body starts utilizing its internal reserves of fats to provide energy. Since there is no glucose that your body has to process, it doesn't need insulin. This, in turn, can help with weight loss.

Intermittent fasting also has a positive effect on the secretion of human growth hormone or HGH. HGH helps regulate your body's metabolism, facilitates muscle and bone development, and also regulates your body's composition. The production of HGH reduces with age. By following intermittent fasting, you can improve the levels of HGH in your body, which in turn helps improve your overall health.

Intermittent fasting increases the production of noradrenaline. This hormone helps to break down the fat cells present in your body. The secretion of this hormone essentially turns your body into a fat-burning machine. Once your body starts burning its internal reserves of fat, you will notice a significant dip in the weighing scales.

Intermittent fasting also induces your body into a state of ketosis. Ketosis is not only a desirable process but also a healthy state of metabolism. When your body starts running out of glucose, it dips into its internal fat reserves to provide energy. When your body starts burning fat, it produces ketones. These ketones are used to provide energy instead of glucose. This process is referred to as ketosis. The best way to induce ketosis is by fasting.

Benefits of Intermittent Fasting

Intermittent fasting is certainly a beneficial diet, and the benefits it offers go beyond weight loss. In this section, you'll learn about the different benefits of intermittent fasting.

Better Functioning of Cells

As mentioned in the previous section, there are different changes that take place in your cells when you opt for intermittent fasting. Intermittent fasting helps trigger autophagy. Autophagy is the process of cellular repair. During this state, your body starts to remove any damaged cells and replaces them with healthier and new cells. Apart from this, autophagy also helps in the removal of any toxins building up within. Think of autophagy as your body's housekeeping and maintenance service. Intermittent fasting also causes changes in the levels of certain hormones like insulin. When the level of insulin in your body decreases, it enables your body to start burning fat for providing energy. As mentioned in the previous section, it helps trigger the release of human growth hormone. HGH helps in the development of lean muscle.

Weight Loss

Perhaps one of the most popular reasons why a lot of people opt for intermittent fasting is that it helps in weight loss. While following any of the methods prescribed by intermittent fasting, you don't have to worry about the number of calories you eat. When you start fasting, your food intake decreases, provided you don't try to compensate for it by overeating. For instance, let us assume that you're used to eating three meals along with a couple of snacks between meals. Now, if you start following the 16/8 method, the number of meals you eat will be lessened, so your calorie intake will also decrease. If you want to lose weight, you must ensure that your body maintains a calorie deficit. A calorie deficit occurs when your body's calorie expenditure is greater than the calorie intake. Apart from this, intermittent fasting also helps your body to start burning fat. So you will lose not only weight but also fat.

INTERMITTENT FASTING FOR WOMEN

As mentioned in the previous section, your body has internal reserves of fat. Most of the fat is deposited between organs and beneath the skin. When you start following the protocols of intermittent fasting, your body starts to get rid of this fat. Also, most of the fat present in our body is concentrated in the abdominal area. If you want a flat tummy, intermittent fasting can help you attain that goal.

Combats Type 2 Diabetes

One of the most common health problems that humanity is fighting today is type 2 diabetes. A poor diet, combined with a sedentary lifestyle, is one of the reasons for an alarming increase in type 2 diabetes. You can reduce your risk of exposure to type 2 diabetes and also manage this condition by following intermittent fasting. Whenever you eat something, there will be a spike in your blood sugar levels. When this happens, your body starts producing insulin to counteract the effect of blood sugar. Insulin is secreted by the pancreas, and it helps to regulate blood sugar levels. If your blood sugar level increases, the production of insulin increases too. After a while, your body starts becoming resistant to insulin. When this happens, it becomes quite difficult for your body to process the blood sugar present within. This is the leading cause of diabetes. You can effectively reverse the situation by following the protocols of intermittent fasting. Diabetes is considered to be a risk marker for several cardiovascular disorders. So by effectively managing diabetes, you can reduce your risk of cardiovascular diseases too.

Reduces Inflammation

Your body's first line of defense against any infection is inflammation. Inflammation is desirable in regulated levels. However, when left unchecked, inflammation can become a severe and painful condition. Whenever any unstable molecules start harming any essential proteins like DNA molecules within your body, it causes inflammation. Inflammation is believed to be the primary cause of several painful and chronic health conditions like arthritis. When left unchecked, it causes your body to start attacking itself from within. All this is caused by oxidative stress. Intermittent fasting helps to reverse and prevent oxidative stress. This, in turn, helps reduce inflammation. Oxidative stress is believed to increase the risk of several neurodegenerative disorders. So by tackling inflammation, you can improve your overall health.

A Healthier Heart

For a couple of decades now, there has been an alarming increase in the spread of cardiovascular diseases. Most of this is because of improper eating habits and the sedentary lifestyle we're leading these days. Intermittent fasting helps to regulate different health markers that are associated with cardiovascular disorders. Intermittent fasting can effectively help to reduce your blood pressure. It can also control cholesterol levels and sugar levels. A combination of all these factors means that you will have a healthier heart.

Flexibility

A great thing about intermittent fasting is that it offers flexibility. Unlike a lot of other diets that a rather restrictive, intermittent fasting is very flexible. Not only is it flexible, but it also gives you the chance to customize the diet according to your needs. Since there are no hard and fast rules about when you must fast, you are free to design your day according to your needs. According to your daily schedule, you can select a dieting protocol that fits in very well. Also, it doesn't place any dietary restrictions per se since you have complete autonomy over when you want to fast and how you want to fast, though the likelihood of sticking to this diet in the long run increases.

Simple to Follow

Since there are no dietary restrictions prescribed by this diet, it is quite easy to follow. You don't have to worry about splurging on any expensive ingredients or any nutritional supplements. Intermittent fasting is a diet that oscillates between eating and fasting. As long as you stick to the fasting schedule, you are good to go. If you make it a point to eat healthy and wholesome meals and fast regularly, you will see an improvement in your overall health in no time. Since you don't have to worry about any meal prep or search for any specific recipes, it becomes easier to follow this diet. Apart from this, there are plenty of intermittent-fasting-friendly recipes that are given in this book that will come in handy while following this diet.

Sustainability

A wonderful thing about intermittent fasting is that it is sustainable in the long run. A lot of fad diets that prescribe crash dieting or extreme food restrictions aren't sustainable in the long run. If you cannot stick to a specific diet for more than a couple of weeks, you might start gaining all the weight you managed to lose. Since this diet doesn't deprive you of any specific food groups, it certainly is sustainable in the long run.

Side Effects to Watch Out For

Well, intermittent fasting certainly has different health benefits. Changing your diet is a major change your body has to undergo. So it will take your body some time to get used to the new diet. In the meanwhile, you can experience specific side effects. However, you don't have to worry about the side effects because they can be managed. In this section, you will learn about certain potential side effects along with how you can manage them.

Hunger

One of the common side effects that you will notice when you change your diet is hunger. If you like to snack, it can be a little tricky once you start following intermittent fasting. Most of us are used to eating maybe five or even six times a day. Since you are used to this, your body starts to expect food at specific times. In such instances, your body produces ghrelin. Ghrelin is a hormone that regulates hunger. Once you start following any of the protocols of intermittent fasting, the frequency of your meals will be lessened. This means that you will begin experiencing hunger pangs. These hunger pangs usually go away in a week or so after your body gets used to the diet. You can also tackle hunger by ensuring that you fill yourself up with nutrient-dense foods whenever you eat. If you feel full, your desire to eat will decrease. Also, make it a point to keep drinking plenty of water. You will learn about more tips on managing hunger in the subsequent chapters.

Headaches

If your diet is predominantly made up of carbs and processed foods, your body will need some time to get used to the new diet. The same stands true if you are used to constant snacking. One of the common symptoms you will experience while your body gets used to the new diet is a mild headache. Headaches can also be caused due to stress and dehydration. So by drinking plenty of water and electrolytes, you can prevent dehydration.

Cravings

If you're making any dietary changes, you can experience certain cravings. For instance, if you are told that you can never eat cupcakes, you start craving cupcakes. It is basic human psychology that you start craving for something when you're told that you can't have it. So a simple way to prevent this is by making sure that you don't deprive yourself of any food for starting this diet. All you must do is make a healthy and conscious choice about the food you eat. By avoiding or limiting your intake of junk food, you can attain this objective. Try to fill yourself up with nutrient-rich foods so that you feel fuller for longer. If your tummy is full, any cravings you experience will decrease. Since there are no dietary restrictions, maybe you can come up with healthier alternatives to the foods you love.

Low on Energy

Your body will need a while to get used to intermittent fasting. It can take anywhere between a week to 10 days for your body to get acclimatized to intermittent fasting. By opting for this diet, you are essentially changing the primary source of energy in your body. This can make you feel tired or sluggish. Once you get used to this diet, your energy levels will go up. Also, it is a good idea to avoid any high-intensity exercises during the first couple of weeks of fasting. Be patient with your body and give it the time it needs to get used to the new diet.

Irritability

Experiencing hunger pangs or even being low on energy can make you quite irritable. A drop in your blood sugar levels can also cause irritability, so ensure that you give your body all the nutrients it needs and make sure that you are thoroughly hydrated. By doing this, you can reduce your irritability. Also, start concentrating on doing such things that make you happy while avoiding anything that's stressful.

Urge to Overeat

The eating window will be significantly reduced once you start following this diet. Since you no longer can eat all day long, you might feel like overeating within the given time frame. You might have the urge to binge on unhealthy foods the minute you break your fast. However, prevent yourself from doing this. A simple tip that you can use is to ensure that you consume plenty of wholesome and nutrient-dense foods before you feel like eating any unhealthy junk. Once you are full, the urge to overeat will also decrease.

The benefits that this diet offers certainly outweigh any possible side effects. You might or might not experience the different side effects discussed in this section. However, by being aware of these things, you can take steps to prevent them or reduce their intensity.

CHAPTER 3: METHOD OF INTERMITTENT FASTING

Different Methods

Intermittent fasting (IF) is one of the most popular dieting protocols these days. One of the main reasons for its popularity is the flexibility it offers. Unlike other diets, intermittent fasting provides different dieting protocols, and you can select one according to your lifestyle needs and fitness goals. In this section, you will learn about the different methods of intermittent fasting.

16/8 Method

One of the easiest forms of intermittent fasting is the 16/8 method. Your body is essentially fasting whenever you're asleep. Given the daily diets that we are used to, the only period we all fast are while we are sleeping. This method of intermittent fasting is a mere extension of the fasted state your body is in while asleep. If you are habituated to skipping breakfast, eating the first meal in the afternoon and your last one at night, then you are fasting for around 16 hours a day. When you do this, the eating window is restricted to about 8 hours. Precisely, this is what you are required to do while following this protocol. You can plan out your day according to your convenience. The only principle of the 16/8 method is that you are required to fast for 16 hours and have an eating window to 8 hours. You can easily eat three meals and maybe even a snack during this window.

For instance, if your first meal is at noon and your last one at 8:00 p.m., then you successfully fasted for 16 hours. It does sound quite simple, doesn't it? This method is rather convenient for anyone who doesn't like eating breakfast in the morning. When you skip a meal and reduce the eating window, you are inadvertently limiting your calorie intake too. When you do this, your body starts burning fat to provide energy during the fasting period. All of these factors assist in weight loss. As mentioned earlier, you can customize this diet according to your needs. If you like waking up in the morning and maybe exercise a little, adjust the eating window accordingly. Maybe you can have your first meal at 10:00 a.m. and your last one at 6:00 p.m. As long as you fast for 16 hours on a given day, you are good to go.

The 5:2 Diet

If the thought of fasting every day doesn't appeal to you, don't worry because intermittent fasting has different methods, and at least one will fit your lifestyle. The principle of the 5:2 diet is quite simple. You are required to fast for two days a week and eat like you normally do on the other days. On the days of the fast, you can eat as long as your calorie intake doesn't exceed 500 to 600 calories. You're free to choose the two days of the week that you want to fast on. The only thing you must keep in mind while doing this is to ensure that you don't fast on two consecutive days. For instance, if you start your fast on Monday, then the next day you must fast on will be Wednesday. Don't worry about the calorie restriction because you can still eat two or even three light meals. As long as you don't try to compensate for the fasting days by stuffing yourself with unhealthy junk on the other days of the week, you will see an improvement in your overall health.

Even if you fast for just two days a week, you can speed up the process of weight loss. On normal days, make sure that you eat healthy and wholesome foods. The calorie restriction for men and women is 600 and 500 calories, respectively.

The Warrior Diet

This protocol of intermittent fasting doesn't prescribe a strict fast. You are free to consume raw fruits as well as vegetables during the day in small amounts. At the end of the day, you are free to eat a hearty meal. You are mainly required to fast throughout the day and feast at night. By following this protocol, you will notice that the eating window is restricted to just about four hours a day.

This dieting protocol is a perfect combination of intermittent fasting and the Paleo diet. The Paleo diet refers to a method of eating wherein you are required to eat like our ancestors used to back in the Paleolithic era. It essentially means that you cannot consume any processed carbs or sugars. While following this diet, you can eat plenty of fruits, vegetables, and animal protein. If you aren't sure what you can and cannot eat, here is a simple solution. If something looks like it wouldn't have been accessible to our caveman ancestors, then you cannot eat it. Anything that looks like it was produced in a factory is strictly off-limits while following this diet. You will be following a high-fat and a low-carb diet. So you are required to stay away from all carbs and starchy foods. Instead, fill yourself up with naturally fatty protein along with plenty of fruits and vegetables.

Spontaneous Fasting

Well, this method of fasting is precisely what the name suggests. You are required to fast spontaneously. There is no prior planning or preparation required. Whenever you don't feel like eating, simply skip a meal. It is as simple as that. At times, we tend to get quite busy with work or might not have the appetite for a meal. In such instances, don't eat. Eat only when you are hungry and not because you have too. By skipping a couple of meals every week, you can effectively reduce your calorie intake. This method of fasting will help you become attuned to the needs of your body. Don't worry that your body will shift into starvation mode if you skip your meals. As long as you have a healthy and balanced diet, you're nothing to worry about.

The Eat-Stop-Eat Protocol

In this method of intermittent fasting, you are required to fast for 24 hours. You can either fast once or twice a week and not more than that. While deciding the fasting days, ensure that they are not consecutive. For instance, if you had your dinner at 7:00 p.m. on Monday, you are required to fast until 7:00 p.m. on Tuesday. If you keep fasting on two consecutive days, you might shift your body into starvation mode. Once your body shifts into this state, it will stop burning fats.

While fasting, you are prohibited from consuming any solid food. However, you can consume plenty of calorie-free beverages along with any other intermittent fasting friendly. If weight loss is your primary objective, make sure that you are consuming healthy and wholesome meals when you are fasting. Perhaps the only tricky part about this method of fasting is that you are required to fast for 24 hours at a stretch. It might not be easy to start following this method initially. However, once you get used to fasting, it will come naturally. It is a good idea to start with any of the previous methods of intermittent fasting and then slowly make your way to this protocol.

How to Select a Method of Fasting

Now that you are aware of the different forms of intermittent fasting, you must select one. The method you select is quite essential. The success of sticking to the diet depends on the method you choose. If you opt for a technique that keeps clashing with your schedule and daily lifestyle, it is unlikely that you will stick to it in the long run. There are three simple steps that you must follow while selecting a dieting protocol, and they are as follows:

What Do You Feel about Fasting?

Any diet is certainly a change. Change is never easy, but it is essential. When it comes to following a diet, you must ensure that you are thoroughly invested in it. If you want to stick to your diet in the long run, regardless of the method of intermittent fasting you opt for, you must ensure that you're comfortable with it. So take a moment and think about what your personal opinion is about fasting. If you don't like the idea of fasting or having a fasting schedule, then the chances of following this diet will dwindle down. If you want to try a new diet, you must keep an open mind about it and embrace the unique experience. You must maintain a positive attitude toward intermittent fasting if you want this diet to be successful.

What Is Your Daily Schedule?

Intermittent fasting is not a complicated diet. It offers a lot of flexibility, and there are different methods of fasting. While selecting an ideal method of fasting, you must ensure that it doesn't clash with your daily schedule. If a diet clashes with your regular schedule, it is quite likely that you will end up giving up on it. For instance, if you don't like having breakfast in the morning and are signed with the idea of fasting for 16 hours a day, then you can opt for the 16/8 method.

If you are not used to having any meals during the day and instead like to have some snacks and end your day with a heavy meal, you can opt for the warrior diet. If you select the diet that fits in perfectly with your lifestyle and your daily schedule, the chances of success increase. Understand that any diet you opt for must not be a cause of additional stress. If your diet seems stressful to you, you will lose the motivation to keep going.

What Is Your Usual Diet?

Is your usual diet mainly made up of carbs, sugars, or other processed foods? If yes, then transitioning to intermittent fasting might be a little tricky. You might not have realized it, but a diet that is rich in carbs and sugars is rather addictive for your body. So making any changes to such a diet will take some time and effort. If you want to follow any method of intermittent fasting, such as the eat-stop-eat method or the 16/8 method, you must prepare yourself to fast for extended periods. While doing this, it is quite natural to experience sugar withdrawal. Remember that your body has been conditioned to a particular diet and is used to eating at specific times. When you start fasting, you are fundamentally shifting your body into a fasted state from a continuously fed state. So it is but natural that you will experience sugar withdrawal. However, this isn't a reason not to start a new diet. There are certain tips you can take to make this process of transition easier on yourself.

The first step is never to select a dieting protocol that is too stringent or strict for your body. There is no rush, and you can take the time your body needs to get used to the diet. Start working slowly to ensure that your body gets used to intermittent fasting. For instance, you can start by removing certain kinds of carbs from your daily diet. You can start eliminating one type of carb from your diet every other day. By doing this, you are slowly conditioning your body to a new diet. Once you start following any of the protocols of intermittent fasting, you will not experience symptoms of withdrawal. Apart from this, it will also make it easier to start making healthier food choices.

If you like snacking between meals and are used to snacking constantly, start increasing the gap between two meals. For instance, if you're used to having a snack between breakfast and lunch, start avoiding it. Once you start filling yourself up with healthy and wholesome foods, you will feel fuller for longer. By doing this, it will reduce your urge to snack. Once you do away with snacking all together, it becomes easier to fast.

Take some time and think about these three steps. Carefully consider what you can and cannot do. Once you do this, you will have your answer!

CHAPTER 4: ABOUT AUTOPHAGY

What Is Autophagy and How Does It Work?

Did you know that your body tends to eat itself? Yes, it does, and there is nothing unnatural about it. It might sound a little scary, but it is good. Autophagy is a process wherein your body starts to clean itself from within by getting rid of any toxins or damaged cells. It enables the creation of healthy and new cells, as well as the repair of any damaged cells. Various dead cells, proteins, and other oxidized particles tend to accumulate in your cells over time. All these undesirable cells hinder the internal mechanism of your body. This accumulation of toxins speeds up the process of aging, increases the risk of certain cancers, induces dementia, and prevents your body from functioning optimally. A lot of cells present in your body, especially the ones in your brain, must last you a lifetime. So your body has created a unique system that helps you to get rid of any damaged cells and defend it from any diseases. Autophagy is a natural defense mechanism that ensures that your body is functioning optimally.

Does this sound a little too complicated? Well, here is a simple analogy that will make things clearer. Your body is like a car. After you drive your car for certain miles, you need to get it serviced. If you don't get it serviced from time to time, your car doesn't perform like it's supposed to. The oil needs to be changed. The coolant has to be replaced. The tires need to be filled with air. And there are many other damages that need to be fixed. This is how autophagy works in your body.

Now, let us take the same situation. However, this time, you are older and not as efficient as you once used to be. After using your car for a while, you might not get it serviced. You might forget about monthly maintenance or ignore any troubles your car is giving. Any damage that your car has sustained hasn't been repaired. All this means that your car will not function optimally. This is what happens when autophagy isn't working as it's supposed to in your body. Autophagy is a process that usually works in the background to help with the regular upkeep of your body. It is usually triggered in a high-stress situation. Since it is your body's defense mechanism to any diseases, it is automatically triggered whenever your bodies under any duress. By doing this, it improves your body's ability to tackle any illnesses and improves the functioning of all the internal cells.

Detox diets, as well as juice cleanses, have become rather popular these days. However, they are fad diets, and like any fad, even they will fade away slowly. Having a kale smoothie to detox your body is perfectly fine. There is a better way to get rid of all toxins from your body. The human body is capable of cleansing itself from within. The good news is that you have complete control over this process. To trigger this process, you need to enable your body to cells cannibalize. It might sound a little scary, but it is a natural process. You can start training your body to cannibalize itself. This process is known as autophagy, and as mentioned, it detoxifies your body. There are plenty of damaged and dead cells within your body, so you need to enable your body to remove all of these useless cells to improve its functioning.

When autophagy is triggered, it encourages your body to gobble up any damaged cells and replace them with new ones. To make sure that your car is functioning, you must send it for servicing. Likewise, your body also needs autophagy.

The scientific term for autophagy is *autophagocytosis*. Autophagy places your body on a recycle mode where it starts to get rid of all the waste that's been piling up within. Autophagy essentially places your body in a *catabolic state*, which helps process tissues, instead of the *anabolic state*, which encourages tissue formation. There are different benefits that autophagy offers. It helps to strengthen your immune system while reducing inflammation. It also helps to slow down the process of aging and encourages the removal of cancerous cells or tumors from the body. Apart from this, it also removes any toxins or infectious substances present in your body. The lack of autophagy can increase your cholesterol and induce laziness. It can also lead to obesity and brain impairment.

Now, let us learn about the way autophagy works in your body. When autophagy is triggered, all the cells present in your body start to look for any dead or malfunctioning cells. Once the cells are identified, they are destroyed. Technically, the cells are destroyed, but the healthy cells consume them. The healthy cells create a double membrane around the unhealthy cell, and it is referred to as an autophagosome. The unhealthy or toxic cell is then devoured by the autophagosome. This, in turn, produces energy. So how is autophagy regulated in your body?

Are you wondering how intermittent fasting helps to trigger autophagy? Autophagy is triggered whenever there is a calorie deficit, which happens when your energy expenditure is more than your calorie intake. When there is a calorie deficit, it encourages the healthy cells in your body to start removing any unnecessary proteins. All such damaged cells are broken down and converted into amino acids, which provide your body with energy.

The benefits provided by intermittent fasting are because of autophagy. Being in a fasted state triggers autophagy. When your body is in a fasted state, it starts using its energy reserves to supplement your body's energy requirement. If you keep supplying it with fuel, it will not utilize any fats stored within. Your body is kicked out of autophagy whenever you consume any calories. So by following intermittent fasting, you enable your body to cleanse itself.

For instance, if you are following the 16/8 method of intermittent fasting, your body is in a fasted state for about 16 hours a day. It takes your body anywhere between six to eight hours to digest the food you consume. Only when this food is digested will it shift into a fasted state. Essentially, your body isn't in a fasted state until six hours into the fasting period. As mentioned earlier, autophagy keeps running in the background. However, if you keep your body in a fed state, then autophagy isn't effective. Your body needs to be in ketosis to trigger autophagy. Once this process starts, your body starts to cleanse itself from within. However, you don't have to starve yourself to achieve autophagy. If you shift your body into starvation mode, it will do you no good. Once your body is in starvation mode, it shuts down all functions except the vital ones. Your body will start holding on to any calories present, and it will prevent any unnecessary expenditure. This means it will stop burning any fats and will try to conserve energy.

How to Induce Autophagy?

Autophagy is induced when your body is under stress. Either this or you must consume certain foods that can help trigger autophagy.

There are various ways in which you can trigger autophagy. Since it is your body's natural response to stress, you can trick your body into believing that it's under some stress. In this section, you will learn about how you can induce autophagy.

Aerobic Exercise

You can trigger autophagy in all the tissues present in the brain, along with other muscles in the body with aerobic exercises. Exercise is stress-inducing for the cells in your body. So it helps trigger autophagy. Apart from this, if you exercise, your body will produce endorphins, which will elevate your mood. Regular exercise can improve your overall fitness while speeding up the process of weight loss. Physical exercise is one of the easiest ways to trigger autophagy. Any form of HIIT (high-intensity interval training) triggers autophagy. The stress, which is induced by HIIT, triggers autophagy without harming your muscles. About 20 to 30 minutes of HIIT twice or thrice per week will do the trick.

Intermittent Fasting

Any diet that encourages calorie restriction the way intermittent fasting does can trigger autophagy. Whenever there is a shortage of glucose in the body, autophagy is activated. It helps recycle any toxic waste that's present within and gets rid of damaged cells to make more room for healthy cells. Abstaining yourself from food for short periods can help. Short-term fasts prescribed by intermittent fasting will certainly come in handy. When you fast, your body starts to believe that it is under some form of stress and activates autophagy as its first line of defense.

Sleep Is Essential

It is quintessential that you get at least seven hours of undisturbed sleep every night. Sleep has a therapeutic effect on your body. It not only enables your body to function optimally but also regulates the circadian rhythm. Apart from this, autophagy kicks in when you are sleeping. The circadian rhythm helps regulate your sleep cycle and is also related to autophagy. Your circadian rhythm is your body's biological clock. So if it performs optimally, it will trigger autophagy. Also, getting a good night's rest will make you feel refreshed and energetic in the morning.

Restricting Protein

You can trigger autophagy by reducing your protein consumption once or twice per week. Ensure that your protein intake doesn't exceed 10 to 15 grams per day on the days of a protein fast. By doing this, you are encouraging your body to start recycling any proteins present within. This, in turn, helps reduce inflammation while cleansing your cells without any muscle loss. Once autophagy is triggered, your body starts to devour any malfunctioning proteins and starts to get rid of all toxins.

The Ketogenic Diet

A low-carb and high-fat diet like the keto diet encourages your body to start burning fats to provide energy. By changing your body's primary source of energy, you can induce autophagy. Your body undergoes a similar change when you follow the protocols of intermittent fasting. Also, the great thing about the keto diet is that you can easily combine it with the protocols of intermittent fasting.

To trigger autophagy, you either need to exercise or make changes to your diet. By making your body feels like it is under stress, you can trigger autophagy. Also, you can exercise in moderation while following any of the dietary changes to kick-start autophagy.

CHAPTER 5: HOW TO GET STARTED WITH INTERMITTENT FASTING

Steps to Get Started with Intermittent Fasting

Now that you are aware of different methods of intermittent fasting, all that's left fail to do is get started. In this section, you will learn about certain practical steps that you can follow to get started with intermittent fasting.

Choose a Method

Since there are different methods of intermittent for fasting, it is essential that you select one of the plans. The method that you select must suit your daily lifestyle. A lot of people tend to give up on the diet because it tends to clash with their lifestyle or the daily schedule. To avoid this, you must select a method of intermittent fasting that can easily merge with your regular schedule. Carefully go through your different options and take some time, weighing the pros and cons of each of the methods. Then select one that appeals to you. If you like the dieting protocol that you opt for and it doesn't wreak havoc on your social life, the chances of sticking to it will increase.

Do Your Homework

Well, now that you've selected the method of intermittent fasting you wish to follow, it is time to gather all the necessary tools to help you along the way. There are various apps as well as online trackers that you can use to ensure that you are sticking to your diet. When it comes to intermittent fasting, it is a process of trial and error. So you need to keep track of the methods you try along with the foods you consume. You can always maintain a food journal to keep track of the progress you make, the food you eat, and the diet to follow. By making a conscious effort, it becomes easier to stick to intermittent fasting. If you keep doing this for a couple of weeks, it will come to you naturally.

The method that might have seemed to work for someone else might not necessarily work for you. So you need to find a method that will work well for your body. You need to research about the different kinds of food that you can and cannot eat while following this dieting protocol. Well, this book certainly makes it all easy because you don't have to do this. You will learn about the foods that you can and cannot eat while following intermittent fasting in the subsequent chapters. Apart from this, you will also find plenty of healthy recipes that you can follow to cook healthy and delicious food.

Time to Transition

Now that everything is in place, it is time to get started with the diet. Ensure that you start your diet from that day. If you are new to fasting, the thought of going for prolonged periods without food might not appeal to you, so you will need to start conditioning your body to get used to the idea of fasting before you can follow any of the protocols of this diet. For instance, you can slowly start increasing the gap between two meals and avoid stacking. Apart from this, you can start replacing all the unhealthy foods you consume with healthy and wholesome foods. If your tummy stays fuller for longer, you will notice that it isn't difficult to skip snacks in between meals. Instead of opting for a strict protocol like the eat-stop-eat method, it makes the most sense to start with a more straightforward method like the 16/8 method. Start slowly and give your body the time it needs to get used to the new diet.

Your Support System

When it comes to dieting, having your support system can be quite helpful. There will undoubtedly be days when you don't feel like following a diet, and you will want to give up. Or you might simply lose the motivation to keep going. In such instances, your support system will provide you the motivation necessary to keep going. So who will be a part of a support system? Your support system can consist of your loved ones, family members, friends, colleagues, or anyone else that you can think of. Explain why you want to follow the diet and talk about the goals you want to achieve. By explaining your situation to others, it becomes easier for them to understand you. So find a support system before you get started with the diet.

Exercise Routine

As mentioned earlier, your body will need a while to get used to this diet. If you're used to exercising regularly, reduce the intensity of the walkouts during the first couple of weeks of this diet. Your body will need to get used to burning fats instead of waiting for glucose to provide energy. This change in this process cannot happen overnight and will take some time. In the meanwhile, don't exert yourself too much. If you're not used to fasting, then there are certain side effects that you might experience, such as headaches, fatigue, tiredness, or even irritability. A combination of these factors can make exercising quite difficult. So give your body the time it needs to get used to the diet. You don't have to skip exercising altogether. You must tweak your exercising schedule according to the diet you are following. Avoid any high-intensity training during the first two weeks of intermittent fasting. You can stick to low-intensity exercises, yoga, or a basic core workout. Try to reduce the stress on your body. If you push yourself past your body's threshold, you will merely enjoy yourself. If you train too hard or too long while you are fasting, it can injure your muscle health.

Delayed Gratification

There will obviously be times when you feel like eating a lot of things. At such times, the urge to break your fast, eat foods that you are not opposed to, or even give up on your diet can be too difficult to resist. At such instances, simply follow the technique of delayed gratification. Whenever you feel the urge to eat something that you know you must not, take time out. Stop whatever you are doing and start making a note of all the things you want to eat. Once you do this, you are getting the thought of food out of your head. Now that you have a list of foods you feel like eating, tell yourself that you can eat it later. Instead of telling yourself no, you are merely saying, "Not right now." By doing this, you will not feel like you are denying yourself any foods. Since intermittent fasting doesn't have any strict dietary restrictions, you can have a cheat day once in a while. The only thing that you must keep in mind while doing this is to ensure that you don't go overboard.

Nutrient-Dense Foods

If you're new to fasting, then as soon as you break the fast, the urge to binge on unhealthy foods will be quite high. If you are used to a diet that is predominantly made up of carbohydrates and sugars, shifting to any other diet will be difficult. Your body is primarily used to burning glucose to provide energy, so whenever it feels low on energy, it will start craving for carbs and sugars. If you want to attain your weight loss and fitness goals, then it is quintessential that you start consuming foods that are nutrient-dense. Carbs and sugars contain empty calories. Your body doesn't get the nutrients it needs, but your calorie intake increases. So fill yourself up with foods that will leave you tummy feeling fuller for longer. For instance, if you're following the eat-stop-eat protocol, you will need to fast for 24 hours at a stretch. Before starting the fast, you must fill yourself up with foods that can help keep hunger at bay. By making healthy food choices, you can reduce the chances of wanting to binge on unhealthy foods.

Weigh Yourself

Before you get started with this diet, you need to begin maintaining a record of your body weight along with your body measurements. By doing this, you can measure the progress you make once you start following the diet. You can either use an online app or a journal for this purpose. Apart from this, also take a picture of yourself before you get started. There will be times when you might not be interested in sticking to this diet anymore. In such instances, you can look at the picture you took of yourself before the diet. Also, there will be times when you cannot see a change in the weighing scales but your body measurements change.

While getting started with this diet, remember that your body will need transitioning time. During this period, you can affect certain potential side effects of the diet, as mentioned in the previous sections. To prevent any of these things, you need to not only consume healthy and balanced meals but must also keep your body hydrated. Apart from this, try to keep yourself busy during the fasting period, or if possible, you can plan your fasting period such that it includes your sleeping time too.

Practical Tips to Stay Motivated

Well, starting a new diet can be slightly tricky. Did you ever attempt dieting in the past? Are you worried that you might lose your motivation after a couple of weeks? If you want this diet to be effective, you must understand that it isn't a temporary solution. Intermittent fasting is not a quick fix; it is a way of life. If you want to attain your weight loss and fitness goals, you must ensure that your motivation levels don't falter. Motivation can give you the encouragement and motivation to keep going even when you want to give up. In this section, you will learn about the different tips that you can follow to ensure that you stay motivated.

SMART goals

Before you can get started with the diet, it is quintessential that you set certain goals yourself. Ask yourself, Why do you want to follow this diet? What do you plan on achieving from the start? Take some time and answer these questions. Once you have answered these questions, you will most likely have your goal. When you set goals for yourself, it not only becomes easier to measure your success but also gives you the motivation to keep going. However, you must make it a point to set SMART goals. SMART is the acronym used to denote *specific*, *measurable*, *attainable*, *relevant*, and *time-bound* goals. Only when the goal you set meets all these criteria will you be able to achieve them. If you set impractical or unattainable goals yourself, you are merely setting yourself up for disappointment. An example of impractical goals would be to try to lose 10 pounds within a week. When you set a goal like this one, you will only be disappointed with yourself when you cannot attain it. Even if you can achieve it by some means, it is not only unhealthy but can also harm you. An example of a SMART goal would be to lose 20 pounds in 20 weeks. You must not only try to lose weight, but you must try to do so healthily if you want to maintain the weight loss.

Pace Yourself

Your daily schedule, along with your lifestyle, will influence the effectiveness of the diet. If you want to be able to attain your fitness and weight loss goals, you must stick to the diet. The diet will work, but it will take a while. Don't expect to see any miraculous changes overnight. If you want to lose weight and maintain the weight loss, you must stick to the diet. It is not a short-term solution, and it is a lifestyle change. If you want, you always have the option of following one of the crash diets and lose a couple of pounds quickly. However, you will not be able to maintain such weight loss because it isn't sustainable or healthy. If there is a drastic change in your weight, it can cause certain undesirable changes in your body. Intermittent fasting is a brilliant dieting protocol, and it is sustainable. So slow down and understand that there is no rush. You can dictate the pace for yourself. Your body's metabolism, coupled with the dieting protocol you follow, will influence the results you obtain.

Setbacks Are Common

When you are making a major change, you will face a few hurdles. Setbacks are a common part of life. On the journey to success, you will not only have to face setbacks, but you will also have to overcome them. A major reason a lot of people give up on a diet is that they lose motivation as soon as they face an obstacle. You need to change your attitude toward success if you want to stick to your diet in the long run. It is okay to chase perfection but trying to be a perfectionist all the time will bring you nothing but disappointment. For instance, there will definitely be times when you might be tempted to break your diet and eat something that you know you're not used to. Maybe you have a sudden urge to binge on a couple of chocolate chip cookies.

At times, it is okay even if you cannot resist yourself and give in to this temptation. However, the real trouble starts when you start seeing this incident as a major setback. Instead of treating it as a failure, treat it as an isolated incident. Now that you have broken your diet and ate a pint of ice cream or maybe some cookies, don't feel guilty about it. Start the next day, afresh. Temptation can sometimes get the best of you. After all, you are but human. So forgive yourself, and get a clear-eyed view of your goal again. Don't think of one setback as a failure. It isn't a reason and a half to give up on your diet.

Be Patient with Yourself

Remember that your body was used to a certain diet until now. Changing your diet and getting used to a new diet will take some time, so be patient. If you start being impatient with yourself and push yourself too much, you will lose the motivation to stick to the diet. Stick to this diet for at least three weeks if you want to see an improvement. A common challenge that a lot of dieters tend to face is when they have reached a weight loss plateau. There will always come a time when, regardless of what you're doing, the weighing scales don't seem to move. It almost feels like it's stuck. You might be exercising and even following the diet quite carefully. However, you are unable to see a change in the weighing scales. The stage is referred to as the weight loss plateau. At such times, it can be quite difficult to keep up your motivation levels, and you might be tempted to give up.

The first thing that you must do is congratulate yourself for making it this far. Now, all that you need is to make a couple of simple changes to your daily diet. You can start by eliminating all carbs for a while. As soon as you see that you're able to lose weight once again, you can slowly start adding different carbs you eliminated. Give yourself a while to see the way your body reacts to the addition or deletion of certain foods from your diet.

Reward System

You need to create a reward system so that all the efforts you make are acknowledged. You don't need anyone else to acknowledge the fact that you are dieting. But you need to celebrate victories. Now that you are aware of your goals, it is time to break them down into smaller goals. An example of a mini-goal would be to try to follow your diet for 15 days at a stretch without having the cheat day. Or maybe it could be something as simple exercising three times a week. You can come up with your own mini-goals, and it should take you a step closer to your main goal. As soon as you reach one of your many goals, reward yourself. Ensure that the rewards you set are not related to food. Perhaps you can buy yourself the cashmere scarf that you were eyeing for a while. Or maybe even go for a mani-pedi session. As long as the rewards are not food-related, setting up a reward system is a very good idea. By celebrating your achievements, it gives you the motivation to keep going. Whenever you feel a little low on motivation or you feel like giving up on a diet, take a moment and think about all the little goals that you have achieved along the way. You've certainly made it this far, and you can make it all the way to the top too.

Pair Up

Starting the diet is a major change, so if you do it with a partner or a dieting buddy, it will make this change easier. You can pair up with your loved ones, friends, family members, colleagues, or anyone else. By finding yourself a partner, it becomes easier to stick to a new change. Since you see the other person also experience and go through the same things that you are, it gives you the necessary strength to keep going. There will obviously be times when you lose motivation; at such times, your dieting partner will be your support system. Also, if you have a dieting buddy, you will always have someone to go grocery shopping or exercising with and do other diet-related activities. You will be able to connect with others who are in the same situation as you.

When you know that you are not alone and have a support system in place, it makes it easier to keep going. If none of these options appeal to you, you can always talk to your family and explain the reasons why you have opted for this new diet. Talk to them about the importance of attaining your goals and sticking to this diet. Once you do this, it helps create a sense of accountability. Once you feel like you're accountable to someone else, it automatically makes you want to stand by your words. Having a support system in place will keep giving you the support and the strengths that you need to stick to your diet, especially when you feel like giving up.

Well, keep these simple tips in mind to ensure that your motivation levels stay high while following this diet. Following the diet is as much a physical change as a psychological one. If you have the willpower and the motivation to keep going, then your chances of sticking to the diet, in the long run, will substantially increase. So use the steps to pump up your mojo!

CHAPTER 6: WEIGHT LOSS WITH INTERMITTENT FASTING

Maintenance of the Weight Loss

If you want intermittent fasting to help you attain your weight loss goal, there are a couple of things you must understand. Weight loss doesn't occur overnight, and it takes time and a conscious effort. If you want to stay in shape, you need to develop a couple of healthy habits. The first thing you must do is stick to this diet for at least three weeks if you want to see a visible improvement. Make sure that temporary weight loss is not your goals. You need not only to be able to lose weight but also to ensure that you maintain the weight loss as well. Instead of concentrating on temporary weight loss, it is a good idea to work on developing a healthy regime actively. There are plenty of crash diets that can help you lose weight immediately. However, usually, people tend to regain the weight they lost within no time by following these crash diets. This usually happens because they revert to their unhealthy eating habits. By concentrating on intermittent fasting, you can ensure that you're developing healthy and conscious eating habits.

As mentioned earlier, this diet doesn't come along with any dietary restrictions. Keep in mind that this doesn't permit you to eat anything and everything whenever you want. Showing some self-restraint will do you good. You must learn to recognize and control any unhealthy patterns of eating you might have. While following intermittent fasting, you will automatically become aware of the foods you eat. Once your body and mind get used to intermittent fasting, you will automatically start eating better. It will take a while to get there, but you eventually will. A little self-control will certainly go a long way while trying to lose weight.

Don't complicate things. Understand that your diet must not be a reason for additional stress. Intermittent fasting is very flexible, unlike several other diets. Even if you have plans of eating out, you can go ahead and stick to your schedule without worrying about making any changes. A simple thing that you must do is to eat only when you are hungry and to eat until you are full. Don't eat merely because you're used to eating at a specific time. Start listening to your body; it knows what it wants.

By eating when you're hungry, you become conscious of the food you are consuming. If you eat until you are full, you will reduce the chances of overeating. Don't try to compensate for the fasting period by overeating when you break the fast. Your body has a chance to detoxify itself while you're fasting.

You can certainly eat out, but make sure that you don't make it a regular habit of it. While making any social plans or commitments, ensure that you keep your fasting schedule in mind. You don't have to miss out on your life because of your diet. However, it doesn't mean that you take your diet for granted. If you are serious about attaining your fitness and weight loss goals, you need to stick to the dieting schedule. Learn to be patient with yourself and your body. It takes time and conscious effort, so make a commitment to yourself and ensure that you stick to it. Your efforts will certainly pay off. When you start noticing a visible change in your body, it will give you the necessary motivation to keep going.

Regardless of the intermittent fasting protocol that you decide to follow, your calorie intake will automatically reduce. When you skip a couple of meals or when you don't eat as often as you usually do, your calorie intake will be reduced. By coupling this with physical activity, you can increase your body's calorie expenditure. When your calorie expenditure is more than the calorie intake, your body will be in a calorie deficit. When your body is in a calorie deficit, you will lose weight. Moreover, it encourages your body to start burning all the fats that it has stored within. You will not only lose weight but fat too. So by maintaining a calorie deficit, you can ensure that you stay in shape. You need to exercise, but don't overexert yourself. If you overexert yourself, your body will shift into starvation mode. Once your body enters this mode, it starts conserving calories.

If you want to lose weight and maintain the weight loss, there are two simple principles you must keep in mind. The first principle is to be aware of your diet. The second principle is to include regular physical activity. By being mindful of the food you eat and by including regular exercise, you can attain your weight loss and fitness goals.

Practical Tips for Additional Weight Loss

If you want to lose weight, then intermittent fasting will certainly help you achieve this goal. In this section, you will learn about certain tips that you can use to speed up the process of weight loss.

Start Exercising

If you want to lose weight, you must not only concentrate on your diet but also include some form of exercise. You don't necessarily have to go to the gym and exercise. Any sport or any form of physical activity will do the trick. For instance, if you like to dance, why don't you turn your living room into a dance floor? Dance your heart out and burn calories. By exercising, you increase your body's energy expenditure. By intermittent fasting, your calorie intake will decrease, and by increasing your calorie expenditure, you can maintain a calorie deficit. By doing this, you will start losing weight. Include any form of physical activity to your weekly schedule. Exercising for three days a week will do the trick. You can play a sport. Go swimming, running, jogging, or dancing. You can also do yoga or even go to the gym.

Stay Hydrated

Make sure that you drink plenty of water. If you keep your body hydrated, it helps flush out any toxins building up within. Apart from this, it also reduces any potential side effects associated with intermittent fasting. By drinking water, you can ensure that your electrolyte levels stay balanced. Also, this is an effective way to keep hunger pangs away. When you feel hungry, drink a glass of water. Your hunger will go away. Make it a point to drink at least eight glasses of water per day. Carry a water bottle with you wherever you go. If you're bored of drinking regular water, you can add a couple of sprigs of fresh mint leaves or slices of lemon to spruce it up.

Black Coffee

According to some protocols of intermittent fasting, you are not allowed to eat any solid food during the first period. However, you are free to drink any calorie-free beverages. So you can have plenty of black coffee, herbal teas, or other similar beverages without any calories. Well, one thing that you must keep in mind while doing this is to be mindful of your caffeine intake. Consuming too much caffeine can have a diuretic effect on your body. Also, avoid having any caffeinated beverages before going to bed. If you're following the 16/8 protocol of intermittent fasting, you can start your day with a cup of black coffee. The caffeine in it will wake you up and will keep any hunger pangs at bay. Green tea and black coffee also encourage your body to burn more fats.

Healthier Food Choices

A common mistake that a lot of people make when trying to lose weight is that they try to limit their consumption of food. This isn't right, and you need to limit the consumption of certain foods. For instance, it doesn't make any sense to fill yourself up with empty carbs like processed foods. Instead, you can start filling yourself up with healthy and nutrient-dense foods like vegetables. Don't scrimp on vegetables. Make sure that you eat at least one portion of vegetables with every meal that you have. In fact, it is a good idea to ensure that at least 75% of your carb intake comes in the form of vegetables. Two cups of vegetables and maybe about six cups of leafy vegetables will help you lose weight. Not only will these foods leave you feeling full longer, but it will also help your body burn fats. While fasting, the longer that your tummy stays full, the better your chances of keeping hunger pangs at bay.

Stop Fearing Fats

Fats have been wrongly demonized. All naturally fatty foods are good for your body. The main culprit for weight gain is the consumption of carbs. If you want to lose weight, stay away from carbs. Stop being scared of healthy fats and fatty meats. Foods that are naturally fatty are rich in omega-3 oils that are good for your body. Also, they leave you feeling full for longer.

Beware of Hidden Carbs

If you do have to consume any packaged foods, ensure that you carefully read the list of ingredients printed on it. Even those products that claim to be low-calorie or calorie-free tend to contain some form of carbs. In fact, it is a better idea to opt for full-fat products than fat-free ones. For instance, most of the sugar-free products on the market these days contain artificial sweeteners that can ruin your fast. So carefully read the labels before you buy anything. Keep an eye out for any hidden carbs that can sneak up on you.

Track Your Progress

There are several online applications that you can use to track your progress on this diet. If you want, you can also maintain a food journal to keep track of all the foods you eat along with your body measurements. Make it a point to weigh yourself at least once a week. If you stick to this diet for at least three weeks, you will see a positive change in your body. Keep track of all the carbs you consume. The way your body reacts to certain carbs can help you understand the kind of foods that work well with your metabolism. You don't have to keep track of calories while following this diet, except for the 5:2 protocol. However, if you want to, you can track your daily calorie consumption. If you want to maintain a calorie deficit, then doing this will come in handy.

Planning Your Meals

Regardless of the method of intermittent fasting that you decide to follow, you will be aware of your weekly schedule. Since you are aware of your weekly schedule, it becomes easier to plan your meals. Over the weekend, take some time to do the necessary grocery shopping and plan your weekly meals. By doing this, you not only can you reduce your grocery expenditure, but you can also reduce the chances of eating out. If you know that there's food waiting for you at home, the urge to eat out will be reduced. Also, by planning fewer meals, you can make sure that you are eating healthy and nutritious food. It also gives you complete control over the food you are consuming. By doing a little meal prep, it becomes easier to cook. Moreover, it reduces the time you need to spend in the kitchen.

The good news is that there are plenty of healthy and nutritious recipes in this book. By going through that list, you can make a list of groceries you will require. You not only need to make a list but ensure that you stick to it by shopping as well.

Clean Out the Pantry

It is time that you get rid of any unhealthy food or snacks that you have a new pantry. Get rid of any sugary treats, such as cookies, ice cream, cakes, or any other processed foods. Do you remember the saying "Out of sight, out of mind"? Well, this is quite true. If you don't keep looking at all these tempting foods, it becomes easier not to think about them. By reducing your exposure to temptation, it becomes easier to stick to the diet.

Keep Yourself Busy

By keeping yourself busy with your work or any other chores, you can effectively stop your mind from wandering. A busy mind will not have the time to think about your next meal. Apart from this, it also increases your productivity. So on the days of your fast, make sure that you keep yourself busy. Use your time wisely and spend time doing activities that you enjoy.

Protein Is Good

Don't scrimp on protein. Protein is good for your health. It helps fill up your stomach without harming the state of ketosis your body is in. However, don't consume too much protein. Make sure that a majority of your daily calories come from proteins, fruits, natural fats, and vegetables instead of carbs and sugars.

Probiotics Can Help

Did you know that your gut is home to millions of bacteria? These are referred to as the gut microbiome. The gut microbiome helps in better digestion and absorption of the food you consume. If your gut microbiome function optimally, it can speed up the process of weight loss. As with any other living organism, they need food to sustain themselves. By consuming inflammatory foods, such as flour, sugar, dairy, and unhealthy fats, you are effectively destroying your gut microbiome. So by including probiotics, like buttermilk, kombucha, or sauerkraut, you can help the growth of the helpful bacteria.

Mindful Eating

We all tend to lead rather stressful and busy lives. Most of us don't have the time to eat our meals leisurely. However, start practicing mindful eating if you want to lose weight. Mindful eating is the process of focusing on the food that you eat and nothing else while having a meal. Instead of watching TV or using other electronic gadgets, concentrate on the meal you're eating. Don't be in a rush. Take the time, and see what the food you are eating. Notice all the different flavors, textures, and smells of the food. Spend time and enjoy your meal. Make it a point to chew the food before you swallow slowly. When you start practicing mindful eating, you automatically become aware of the food you consume, along with the amount of food you eat. By chewing your food thoroughly before swallowing, you make it easier for your body to digest and absorb the same. By chewing slowly, you can also reduce the amount of food you consume. Your brain takes about 20 minutes to realize when you are full. If you keep stuffing yourself with food, you will not realize when you are full.

By following the simple tips given in this section, you can speed up the process of weight loss. Also, these tips will enable you to start eating healthier.

CHAPTER 7: FOOD LIST

How to Break a Fast

While following intermittent fasting, you must condition your body to fast for extended periods. You need to learn about the ways in which you are supposed to break a fast by following intermittent fasting. In this section, you will learn about certain practices that you can implement to break your fast safely.

Lose the wing-it mentality. You might have different reasons to follow this diet. You might want to improve your overall health, gain lean muscle, and lose weight. Regardless of your reason, there are certain rules and guidelines that you must keep in mind.

There are several changes that your body undergoes while fasting. Your metabolism changes and hormonal changes occur. When you fast, your body enters the state of ketosis. In ketosis, your liver starts producing ketones to burn fats for providing energy. Whenever you fast, you give your body a chance to enter key to assist. So make sure that you don't increase the stress placed on your gut. Excessive stress on the gut can cause inflammation. If you keep eating anything and everything that you want to, inflammation can occur. Inflammation is one of the causes of weight gain.

There are certain foods that you must avoid consuming whenever you break the fast. Eating foods rich in carbs leads to sodium retention in your body. When this happens, you tend to gain weight. Whenever you are fasting, your body starts getting rid of excess water weight, and if you fill yourself up with carbs, anti-diuresis occurs. When your body starts retaining sodium as well as potassium, it causes bloating. Apart from this, it also reduces your energy levels. So you need to ease your body after breaking the fast and prepare it before you start eating anything.

The duration of the fasting period is another factor that you must consider. If you're just coming off a 24-hour fast, you need to be a little more patient with your body than while following the 5:2 fast. Let us assume that you are fasting for about 16 hours a day. You are close to breaking the fast. While fasting, you're free to drink non-caloric beverages, like water, black coffee, and herbal teas. Now, it is time to break the fast. Instead of breaking your fast by bingeing on food, you need to stimulate your digestive system.

Apple cider vinegar has plenty of health benefits. Before you break the fast, consume a little apple cider vinegar. It helps to restore the pH balance in your body and neutralizes any bad bacteria present in the gut. Apart from this, it also helps to stabilize your blood sugar levels. You're free to drink apple cider vinegar even while fasting, but it is a better idea to have a little of this before breaking the fast.

If you don't like the thought of gulping two tablespoons of apple cider vinegar, you can add it to a glass of warm water. You may also add lemon juice, a pinch of cinnamon powder, and sea salt to this concoction. If you don't like the taste of apple cider vinegar, you can forego this one ingredient and drink the rest. Make sure to drink it about 30 minutes before you break the fast. The citric acid from these ingredients stimulates your gut to produce digestive enzymes. We perform a couple of warm-up exercises and stretches before exercising, right? Well, drinking apple cider vinegar has the same effect on your gut.

You can have a little bone broth after consuming the lemon-cinnamon drink. Not only is bone broth tasty, but it is also a superfood that is full of nutrients and electrolytes. By consuming bone broth at the end of your fast, you are preparing your body to absorb the nutrients present in the food you will consume. Since your gut was trying to cleanse itself value of fasting, you need to give it some time to get used to digesting and absorbing the food you consume after breaking the fast.

If your fast extends for over 20 hours, then have vegetable broth or bone broth before you eat other foods. In fact, this is an ideal practice even if you are fasting for about 16 hours a day. You increase the chances of inflammation if you start stuffing yourself with food as soon as you break the fast. You can have vegetables, fish, or bone broth. Add a little cinnamon to any of these broths to improve the secretion of digestive juices in your gut.

Whenever you fast, your body is in a state of ketosis. If weight loss is your primary goal, then consume foods that will help your body stays in ketosis even after the fast ends. So if you want to stay in ketosis, you need to consume a diet that is full of naturally fatty foods and protein. Avoid consuming carbs and sugar to encourage ketosis. Once your body gets used to this state, it turns into an efficient fat-burning machine.

What to Eat When You Are Breaking a Fast?

If you consume foods that are rich in sodium and carbs after breaking the fast, your body starts retaining water. When your body starts retaining water, it leads to weight gain. Since you're trying to avoid this, you need to prevent your body from retaining water. Understand that your body requires insulin for transporting nutrients from one cell to another. However, if there is a drastic spike in your insulin levels, it induces lethargy and drowsiness. Regardless of the intermittent fasting protocol that you want to follow, ensure that the first meal you consume after breaking the fast is low glycemic.

A low-glycemic meal encourages your body to stay in a semi-fasted state for longer. It prevents any drastic fluctuations in your blood sugar levels. Since your body is already burning ketones to provide energy, you don't have to worry about losing any muscle mass. Since you had bone broth before breaking your fast, your body will not resort to self-cannibalization. You can have two eggs, an avocado, and a handful of nuts along with some spinach to break your fast. A low-glycemic meal can also consist of a can of sardines along with some simple salad. Your body can easily digest lean proteins like eggs and fish when compared to red meats, so don't break your fast with red meats. Always opt for lean proteins when you break the fast.

Another option available is to consume fruits to break the fast. Fruits consist of fructose, and your liver can metabolize these sugars. Fructose cannot be used by your body to replace any muscle glycogen. Your liver can store only up to 100 to 150 grams of glycogen at a time. Whenever you fast-forward 24 hours, your body's reserve of glycogen depletes. When your liver store of glycogen is almost empty, consume fruits. Glycogen is depleted whenever you fast or exercise. If you consume more glycogen while the reserves are full, it only leads to the chelation of fat in your body. However, if you want to stay in ketosis longer, then avoid fruits. Fruits contain sugar, and sugar can push your body out of ketosis. If you do want to eat fruits, make sure that you consume those that are rich in fiber instead of sugars—e.g., berries, pears, and apples.

Now, you might be wondering how much you can eat when you break the fast. It is a good idea to consume small meals whenever you break the fast. Try sticking to about 500 calories. You could consume a big meal if you exercised before breaking the fast. While exercising, your body exhausts its internal glycogen reserves, so you need to fill these reserves up again so that it doesn't shift into a self-cannibalization mode.

After the Fast

In this section, you will learn about certain foods that you must include in your diet. These foods will not only encourage weight loss but also ensure that your body gets all the nutrients it needs.

Water

You might not realize it, but drinking water helps the body flush out toxins as well as dissolved fat. Keep hydrated to prevent any side effects associated with a shift in diet. So if you want to keep migraines, fatigue, and nausea away, drink plenty of water. Your body's composition, along with the diet you consume, will influence the amount of water your body needs. However, as a rule of thumb, it is a good idea to drink at least eight glasses of water per day. Make it a point to drink water regularly and in between meals. Before you start eating a meal, drink a glass of water. A simple way to test whether your body is dehydrated or not is by checking the color of your urine. If your pee is pale yellow or clear, it means your body is hydrated. If it is dark yellow, it means you are dehydrated.

Fish

Not only is fish a lean protein, but it also contains plenty of healthy fats. Consuming naturally fatty fish (e.g., sardines, trout, and salmon) ensures that your body gets plenty of omega-3 fatty acids. You can consume 5–8 ounces of fish per day. Omega-3 fatty acids help improve the performance of your brain. Whenever you are buying fish, make sure that you opt for fish caught in the wild instead of factory-farmed ones.

Leafy Vegetables

All cruciferous vegetables contain plenty of fiber and protein, which are quintessential if you want to develop lean muscle and optimize your health. Make sure that you include at least two portions of leafy vegetables to your daily diet. Also, these foods will leave you feeling fuller for longer.

Avocados

Avocados are a superfood and a great source of healthy fats. Not just that, but they can also leave you feeling full for longer. If you want to, you can also break your fast by consuming avocados.

Legumes

Legumes will provide your body with the necessary digestive fiber. Apart from this, they are quite nutritious. Legumes are versatile and can be added to any meal you want. They are also a rich source of protein. By consuming legumes, you give your body the nutrition and energy that it needs. You can easily add legumes to curries, soups, salads, or anything else that you want.

Berries

Berries are a rich source of antioxidants and several vitamins like vitamins A and C. Apart from this, they are also low in calories. There are various berries you can consume, such as raspberries, blueberries, blackberries, strawberries, and cherries. The antioxidants present in berries, along with the different vitamins, help to tackle inflammation while improving the function of your digestive system. Also, berries can help to strengthen your immune system.

Probiotics

If you want to lose weight, make it a point to include certain probiotics to your daily diet. Probiotics help to improve the health of your gut microbiome, reduce inflammation, and restore the balance. Apart from this, it also helps with weight loss. There are different probiotic foods you can consume, such as yogurt, buttermilk, and sauerkraut.

Eggs

Make it a point to include at least two eggs to your daily diet. Eggs are lean sources of protein. They are easy to cook and quite versatile. Apart from this, they are also low in calories. Also, you can break your fast by consuming eggs. Since eggs are low in calories, they enable your body to stay in a semi-fasted state for longer.

Whole Foods

There are various whole foods that you can opt for instead of processed ones. Whole foods contain plenty of dietary fiber as well as nutrients. They also help improve your body's digestion and metabolic functions.

Potatoes

It is a good idea to limit your carb intake when fasting. Whenever you consume carbs, your body is pushed out of ketosis. However, there are certain types of healthy carbs that you can consume, and potatoes are one of these carbs. If you want to include starch in your diet, make sure that instead of flour and processed foods, it is in the form of potatoes. However, don't think that consuming French fries is a good idea. If you want to eat healthily, you must concentrate not only on the foods you consume but also in the way of cooking. For instance, fried foods are never healthy, whereas boiled foods are.

A simple rule that you can keep in mind while following a new diet is to consume foods that are nutrient-dense.

During the Fast

Unless you opt for intermittent fasting protocols like the warrior diet or the 5:2 diet, you cannot consume any food while fasting. Well, the good news is that you are free to consume plenty of calorie-free drinks. In this section, you will learn about a couple of things that you can safely consume during the fast. By including the list of items given in this section, you can ensure that your hunger pangs stay at bay. Once your body is in a fasted state, there are several physiological changes that take place. All these changes help shift your body into a state of ketosis. The longer your body is in ketosis, the more factual your body burn. However, if you want your body to stay in ketosis, then you must abstain from consuming any calories. If you don't consume any calories, then you don't break your fast. So let us look at different foods that you can consume during intermittent fasting. All these foods will help detoxify your body and cleanse your gut from within.

Baking Soda

Baking soda is commonly used in cooking, so it might come as a surprise that you can consume baking soda while fasting. Baking soda helps balance the pH levels in your body. Apart from this, it helps to reduce any fatigue or tiredness you might experience while fasting. You merely need to add a teaspoon of baking soda to a glass of water and drink it while fasting. It also energizes your body. Sodium bicarbonate (baking soda) helps to ensure that your body has sufficient sodium. Ketosis has a diuretic effect on your body, and by consuming sodium bicarbonate, you can restore the electrolyte balance.

Glauber's Salts

If you want to improve your overall health and body's metabolism, consume Glauber's salts. Glauber's salts are also known as sodium sulfate decahydrate. You can consume 5–20 grams of Glauber's salts a day. You merely need to add a teaspoon of salt to a glass of drinking water while fasting. Glauber's salts can help relieve constipation and improve digestion. However, keep in mind that you must not consume more than 20 grams of these salts since they have laxative properties. Excess consumption of Glauber's salts can result in dehydration as well as diarrhea.

Herbal Teas

Consuming herbal teas can help speed up your metabolism and fight off any hunger pangs. There are various herbal teas that you can consume. If you feel extremely tired or experience fatigue after a tiring day at work, then a cup of peppermint tea can reenergize your body. If you have trouble sleeping at night, then having a couple of chamomile tea before going to sleep can improve the quality of your sleep. All herbal teas contain plenty of antioxidants that help to reduce inflammation and improve your digestion. Green tea is perhaps the healthiest of strings you can consume. Green tea can help improve your body's metabolism and ability to burn fats. However, while consuming herbal teas during your fasting window, make sure that you don't add any sugar, honey, or even milk to the tea.

Coffee

Drinking coffee can effectively suppress hunger while you're fasting. The caffeine that is present not only gives your body a good kick of energy but also speeds up the process of burning fats. There are various benefits that coffee offers. For instance, it helps stabilize blood sugar levels and the polyphenol count in your body. However, don't add any sugar or milk to the coffee want to drink. You can add a little stevia to sweeten your drink or even maybe a pinch of cinnamon to add some flavor. If you want to stay in ketosis for longer, then avoid adding any sugar. If you are habituated to drinking instant coffee, then carefully go through the list of ingredients. Hidden calories can effectively disrupt your fast. By drinking coffee, you can manage any hunger pangs. Well, this doesn't mean that you keep drinking coffee all day long. Too much of caffeine can wreak havoc on your body. It increases cortisol levels and can cause headaches. Apart from this, it can also lead to dehydration. So if you love drinking coffee, then ensure that you replace all the electrolytes and water your body loses.

Apple Cider Vinegar

You can consume apple cider vinegar without kicking your body out of the fasted state. Apple cider vinegar is a wonderful salad dressing, but it has several other uses as well. The antibacterial and anti-inflammatory compounds present in apple cider vinegar can improve your overall health. Apart from this, apple cider vinegar also helps to restore the electrolyte balance in your body. Since it contains no calories and plenty of minerals like iron, potassium, and magnesium, it ensures that your body has sufficient electrolytes. It also helps to regulate the pH levels. Drink a glass of water with a tablespoon of apple cider vinegar added to it before breaking your fast. By doing this, you are essentially prepping your body for the food you will consume once the fast ends. Apple cider vinegar also improves the function of your gut microbiome, so it helps improve the function of your digestive system.

You can consume all the beverages mentioned in this section without worrying about ending your fast. These items will also help improve your energy levels and keep hunger pangs away.

Foods to Avoid on the Fast

There are certain foods that you must avoid while following the protocols of intermittent fasting. In this section, you learn about all the foods you must stay away from to improve the effectiveness of this diet.

Commercially Packaged Foods

You must make it a point to stay away from all foods that look like they were produced in a factory. It essentially means that you need to stay away from cookies, chips, chocolate, and other related products. Artificial flavors, along with all the refined sugars present in it, will undo the benefits you reap from fasting. If you want intermittent fasting to be effective, then stay away from processed foods. When you go grocery shopping, make it a point to steer clear of the middle aisle, where all packaged and processed foods are located.

Refined Sugars

If possible, stay away from all sorts of sugary foods. Processed sugars not only wreak havoc on your gut microbiome but also lead to weight gain. When you consume sugar, your body starts using the glucose produced from it instead of using the internal resource of fat. If you want to stay in ketosis, then avoid all sorts of sugary treats.

Alcohol

Did you know that alcohol is a mood depressant? It is a popular misconception that alcohol can make a person happy. However, it produces stress-inducing hormones that can make you feel sad. Also, alcohol leads to inflammation. So if you want to lose weight, then it is a very good idea to stay away from alcohol.

By avoiding the consumption of these foods, you can speed up the process of weight loss. Apart from this, it also helps to ensure that you reap all the benefits provided by intermittent fasting.

Myths about Intermittent Fasting

Intermittent fasting is certainly a very popular dieting protocol. However, there are several myths associated with it. Most of these misconceptions prevent you from attaining your weight loss and fitness goals, and they don't allow your body to reap the benefits of intermittent fasting. By asking these myths, you can speed up the process of weight loss.

Do Not Skip Breakfast

You might have probably heard others say that breakfast is the most important meal of the day. Well, this is a popular misconception.

A lot of people tend to believe that, by skipping breakfast, they increase the chances of weight gain. However, when you take a moment to think about it, you realize that this is wrong. If you skip a meal, your calorie consumption will be reduced. If calorie consumption is reduced, how can you put on weight? So if you don't like eating breakfast or if you are following the pattern of fasting wherein you can't eat breakfast, then you have nothing to worry about. You will not gain weight by skipping breakfast. While you are sleeping, your body burns fats and stores it as energy. So as soon as you wake up in the morning, you usually experience a burst of energy. This energy can keep you going until noon when you have your first meal of the day.

Eating Small Meals

A lot of people believe that eating frequent small meals can help you lose weight. Well, this is another misconception. Let us assume that your total calorie consumption in a day is about 2,000 calories. Now, if you consume these calories in the form of five meals or even three meals, the calorie intake doesn't change. Your body will utilize the same amount of energy to digest and absorb these calories. Also, if you keep consuming food at regular intervals, your body can never stay in a fasted state. If your body isn't in a fasted state, then you cannot reap the benefits offered by intermittent fasting. To keep your body in a fasted state, you must abstain yourself from eating. So don't worry that you need to eat frequently to lose weight. By merely following the protocols of intermittent fasting, you can lose weight.

Constant Snacking

People tend to believe that constant snacking can keep hunger at bay. They also believe that constant snacking prevents the chances of overeating. If you keep eating, you will obviously feel full. However, you don't need to snack constantly to keep yourself feeling full. Whenever you eat, if you consume healthy and wholesome foods, then you will feel fuller for longer. Make it a point to consume plenty of protein, naturally fatty foods, and fibrous foods. A combination of all these things will leave you feeling full for longer. So you don't have to snack constantly. Also, if you keep snacking, your body will keep producing glucose. If this happens, it will never start utilizing its internal resource of fat. If this doesn't happen, you will not lose weight.

You need to maintain a calorie deficit to lose weight. However, it doesn't mean that you need to reduce your calorie intake drastically. Sticking to a strict calorie-restrictive diet will not do your body any favors. In fact, it would have a detrimental effect on your weight loss. Intermittent fasting is quite easy to follow when compared to other restrictive diets. Intermittent fasting reduces your body's response to insulin. Insulin helps in the regulation of blood sugar levels in your body. If you keep providing your body with food, it will keep releasing insulin. If insulin is produced, your body will never start burning fat. So if you want to improve your overall health and lose weight, you need to keep your body in a fasted state.

Nutrient Deficiencies

A lot of people seem to worry that intermittent fasting can lead to nutrient deficiencies. Well, this is a myth as well. As long as you make sure that you are eating healthy and wholesome foods, your body will get all the nutrition that it needs to function optimally. The real trouble starts when you stop consuming healthy foods. If you're worried about any nutrient deficiencies, consult your healthcare provider. There are several multivitamins that you can take to replenish your body with the nutrients it needs. If you follow the food list given in this book, you can ensure that your body doesn't have any nutrient deficiencies.

Loss of Muscle Mass

It is a myth that intermittent fasting leads to muscle loss. Another common misconception is that fasting for extended periods leads to muscle loss. Muscle loss occurs when your body starts to cannibalize itself. This process occurs when your body is in starvation mode. As long as you are fasting and your body is in a fasted state, you've nothing to worry about. If you provide your body with an alternative source of energy to replace the depletion of glycogen, your body will not cannibalize itself. When you're fasting, your body is in a state of ketosis. When in ketosis, your body is constantly burning fats to provide energy.

Eating Disorders

A misconception that needs to be addressed immediately is that intermittent fasting can cause eating disorders. Well, if you have ever heard this, then you have been misinformed. If you stick to any of the protocols of intermittent fasting and eat healthily, it doesn't cause any eating disorders. If you have a history of eating disorders or are recovering from one, then don't attempt this diet.

Athletic Performance

It is a popular misconception that intermittent fasting can have an adverse effect on your athletic performance. If you make any changes to your diet, your body will take a while to get used to these changes. During the transition period, it is quite natural that you might experience low levels of energy. However, it goes away when your body gets used to the new diet. The same applies to intermittent fasting as well. During the initial weeks, while your body is getting used to this diet, you might feel a little tired and even experience fatigue. However, all of this goes away when your body gets used to intermittent fasting. In fact, once your body is used to this diet, you will experience a surge in your energy levels. Since your body is continuously burning fats, you will have a constant source of energy. If you have a constant supply of energy, how will you feel tired? So you don't have to worry about this diet harming your athletic performance. During the first couple of weeks of this diet, it is a good idea to limit your physical activity.

Fertility Issues

A lot of people tend to believe that intermittent fasting also causes fertility issues and women. Intermittent fasting certainly causes changes in different hormones in your body. However, there is no scientific evidence to back the claim that it can cause infertility in women. Well, if you are pregnant, trying to conceive, or are breastfeeding, then it is a good idea not to diet. Your body needs plenty of nutrition during these stages, and if you start reducing your calorie consumption, it can have an adverse effect on your overall health. Intermittent fasting is safe for all healthy adults. Yes, it is true that a woman's body is more sensitive to signals of hunger than a man's body, but it doesn't cause any fertility problems. The real trouble starts when you stop eating healthy foods. If you give your body the nutrition it needs, there's nothing to worry about. As long as your body is in a fasted state and not in starvation mode, you will continue to lose weight.

If you want this diet to be effective, you need to keep an open mind toward it. Don't harbor any of the misconceptions that have been discussed in this section. Intermittent fasting is an effective way to attain your weight loss and fitness goals. If you believe these myths, then it will prevent you from attaining the benefits this diet offers.

Follow IF even while Eating Out

One great thing about intermittent fasting is that you don't have to give up on your social life or even stop eating out. This diet is quite flexible and convenient. You can customize it according to your needs. You don't have to give up on your social commitments because you're following this diet. For instance, if you have to go out with dinner, you can schedule your fasting time accordingly. If you are following the 16/8 schedule and you know that you need to go out for dinner, then you merely need to shift your fasting time to accommodate your plans. You can probably schedule your day such that your fast ends at 9:00 p.m. By doing this, you will not feel like you are giving up on having fun and will be able to stick to the diet too.

Whenever you go out, make a conscious decision about eating healthy. For instance, instead of filling yourself up on the bread basket, you can have plenty of meat and salads. Instead of ordering a big bowl of pasta, you can opt for a grilled steak along with a portion of house salad. It is all about making healthy food choices. It is quite easy to eat out while following this diet. Whenever you are eating out, make sure that you stick to the food list that was discussed in the previous section.

Avoid foods that are rich in sugar and carbs. You can always ask for customized dishes. Ask your waiter if they can make room for your dietary options. Instead of mashed potatoes, you can ask an extra portion of salad. You can also order simple appetizers instead of the main course. For dessert, you can have a little whipped cream with some berries without any sugar. Or maybe you can have a cup of coffee. As long as you're mindful of what you're eating, it is good.

At times, you might feel like giving in to your temptations and end up bingeing on unhealthy treats. If that's the case, don't feel guilty about it later. You can always get back to your diet the next day. The problem starts if you start viewing this as a failure. There are plenty of options regardless of where you go; you just need to look for them. Whenever you are eating out, make it a point to opt for nutrient-dense foods. Fill yourself up with plenty of protein and naturally fatty foods. By doing this, you can ensure that your body stays in ketosis. The longer your body stays in ketosis, the more efficient will it become at burning fats.

CHAPTER 8: BREAKFAST RECIPES

PEACHES AND CREAM OATMEAL SMOOTHIE

Number of servings: 2

Nutritional values per serving:

- Calories: 331
- Fat: 4 g
- Carbohydrates: 46 g
- Protein: 29 g

INGREDIENTS:

- 2 cups frozen peach slices
- ½ cup oatmeal
- 2 cups almond milk
- 2 cups Greek yogurt, preferably peach flavored
- ½ teaspoon vanilla extract

DIRECTIONS:

1. Add all the ingredients into a blender.
2. Blend until smooth.
3. Divide into 2 tall glasses.
4. Serve with crushed ice.

BERRY AND BEET GREEN SMOOTHIE

Number of servings: 2

Nutritional values per serving:

- Calories: 84
- Fat: 1.5 g
- Carbohydrates: 18 g
- Protein: 2 g

INGREDIENTS:

- ¾ cup unsweetened almond milk
- 1 cup chopped beet greens, discard stems
- 3.5 ounces raw beets, peeled and chopped
- 2 tablespoons fresh orange juice
- ¾ cup frozen mixed berries
- 1 small banana, sliced and frozen

DIRECTIONS:

1. Add all the ingredients into a blender.
2. Blend until smooth.
3. Divide into 2 tall glasses.
4. Serve with crushed ice.

COCONUT MANGO SHAKE

Number of servings: 2

Nutritional values per serving:

- Calories: 235
- Fat: 11 g
- Carbohydrates: 29 g
- Protein: 7 g

INGREDIENTS:

- 4 tablespoons chia seeds, soaked in water for 5–6 hours
- 1 teaspoon vanilla extract
- 1 teaspoon flaked coconut (optional)
- 2 cups coconut milk
- 1 cup frozen mango

DIRECTIONS:

1. Add all the ingredients into a blender.
2. Blend until smooth.
3. Divide into 2 tall glasses.
4. Serve with crushed ice.

OAT AND HEMP SEED SMOOTHIE

Number of servings: 2

Nutritional values per serving:

- Calories: 105
- Fat: 3.2 g
- Carbohydrates: 17.3 g
- Protein: 3.3 g

INGREDIENTS:

- 1 cup pitted fresh cherries, plus extra to garnish
- ¼ cup rolled oats
- 2 teaspoons hemp seeds
- 1 cup almond milk
- Ice cubes, as required

DIRECTIONS:

1. Add all the ingredients into a blender.
2. Blend until smooth.
3. Divide into 2 tall glasses.
4. Serve garnished with cherries.

STRAWBERRIES AND CREAM OATMEAL

Number of servings: 2

Nutritional values per serving:

- Calories: 97
- Fat: 1 g
- Carbohydrates: 18 g
- Protein: 5 g

INGREDIENTS:

- 1 cup old-fashioned oats
- 1 cup chopped strawberries, fresh or frozen, thawed
- 4 tablespoons Greek yogurt
- 2 teaspoons honey
- 2 cups water
- 2 teaspoons ground cinnamon
- 2 teaspoons balsamic vinegar
- 1 teaspoon pure vanilla extract

DIRECTIONS:

1. Add oatmeal, water, and cinnamon into a saucepan. Place the saucepan over medium heat.
2. Cover with a lid. When it begins to boil, lower heat and cook until dry.
3. Meanwhile, add vinegar and strawberries into a bowl. Mash

the strawberries with a fork.

4. Stir in vanilla, yogurt, and honey. Pour into the saucepan (after the oatmeal is dry). Mix well.

5. Cook for a minute. Turn off the heat.

6. Serve in bowls.

OATMEAL WITH PEACHES, CRANBERRIES, AND WHITE CHOCOLATE

Number of servings: 4

Nutritional values per serving:

- Calories: 304
- Fat: 8 g
- Carbohydrates: 53 g
- Protein: 7 g

INGREDIENTS:

- 4 cups almond milk
- 2 teaspoons pure vanilla extract
- 3 tablespoons dried cranberries
- Zest of a lemon, grated
- 2 cups old-fashioned oatmeal or steel-cut oats
- 3 tablespoons peaches, chopped and dried
- 2 tablespoons white chocolate chips

DIRECTIONS:

1. Add milk, vanilla, oatmeal, and dried fruit into a saucepan.
2. Place the saucepan over low heat. Cover and cook until dry. Stir frequently.
3. Turn off the heat. Add lemon zest and white chocolate chips and mix well.
4. Spoon into 4 bowls and serve.

POMEGRANATE-PISTACHIO GREEK YOGURT PARFAIT

Number of servings: 2

Nutritional values per serving:

- Calories: 393
- Fat: 16.8 g
- Carbohydrates: 29 g
- Protein: 31 g

INGREDIENTS:

- 2 cups plain 2% Greek yogurt
- Seeds of 1 pomegranate
- 1 teaspoon pure vanilla extract (optional)
- 80 raw pistachios, chopped

DIRECTIONS:

1. Add yogurt and vanilla extract into a bowl and whisk well.
2. Divide into 4 bowls.
3. Divide equally the pomegranate and pistachio nuts and place over the yogurt.
4. Serve.

GARLIC-MUSHROOM FRITTATA

Number of servings: 8

Nutritional values per serving (using egg whites and olive oil):

- Calories: 108
- Fat: 5 g
- Carbohydrate: 4 g
- Protein: 12 g

INGREDIENTS:

- 8 eggs or 16 egg whites
- ½ cup grated Parmesan cheese
- 20 medium-sized mushrooms, preferably cremini mushrooms
- 1 red onion, chopped
- 4 tablespoons milk
- 4 cups shredded spinach
- 2 teaspoons garlic powder
- 2 tablespoons olive oil or 1 cup broth
- Salt and pepper to taste

DIRECTIONS:

1. Place a skillet over medium heat. Then add oil and heat. Add spinach and mushrooms and sauté for 3–4 minutes.

2. Add garlic powder and sauté for a minute until aromatic. Turn off the heat.

3. Transfer into a round baking dish.

4. Add whites, milk, salt, and pepper into a bowl and whisk well. Pour into the baking dish. Add cheese and stir until well combined.

5. Bake in a preheated oven at 350 °F for 30–45 minutes or until set.

6. Cut into 8 wedges and serve.

TURKEY BREAKFAST SKILLET

Number of servings: 4

Nutritional values per serving:

- Calories: 556
- Fat: 32 g
- Carbohydrates: 9.2 g
- Protein: 65.2 g

INGREDIENTS:

- 2 pounds ground turkey
- 12 organic eggs
- 2 cups salsa

DIRECTIONS:

1. Place a skillet over medium heat. Add oil and heat. Add turkey and cook until brown.
2. Stir in salsa and cook for a couple of minutes.
3. Break eggs at different spots on top of the turkey.
4. Cover and cook the eggs to the desired doneness.

TOFU SCRAMBLE WITH TOMATO AND POBLANO PEPPER

Number of servings: 2

Nutritional values per serving:

- Calories: 182
- Fat: 10 g
- Carbohydrate: 11 g
- Protein: 13 g

INGREDIENTS:

- 8-9 ounces extra-firm, water-packed tofu, drained
- 1 fresh poblano chili pepper, deseeded, chopped (about ¼– ½ cup)
- 1 clove garlic, minced
- ½ tablespoon olive oil
- ¼ cup chopped onion
- ½ teaspoon chili powder
- ¼ teaspoon dried oregano, crushed
- ½ tablespoon lemon juice
- A handful fresh cilantro sprigs (optional)
- ¼ teaspoon ground cumin
- Salt to taste
- 1 plum tomato, deseeded and chopped (about ½ cup)

DIRECTIONS:

1. Place the tofu over paper towels. Dry the tofu by patting with some more paper towels. Crumble and set aside.

2. Place a nonstick skillet over medium-high heat. Add oil and heat. Add poblano pepper, garlic, and onion and sauté for 2–3 minutes.

3. Stir in oregano, chili powder, cumin, and salt. Sauté for a few seconds until aromatic.

4. Add tofu and stir.

5. Lower the heat and cook for 3–4 minutes. Stir occasionally. Turn off the heat.

6. Add tomatoes and lemon juice and mix well.

7. Sprinkle cilantro on top and serve.

BREAKFAST STUFFED SWEET POTATOES

Number of servings: 4

Nutritional values per serving:

- Calories: 179
- Fat: 8 g
- Carbohydrates: 15 g
- Protein: 11 g

INGREDIENTS:

- 2 medium sweet potatoes
- 4 slices center-cut bacon
- 4 large eggs
- ½ cup shredded 2% cheese
- Salt and pepper to taste

DIRECTIONS:

1. Prick the sweet potatoes with a fork all over. Place in the microwave and cook on high for 5 minutes. Turn the sweet potatoes after about 2–3 minutes of cooking.
2. Remove from microwave and place on your cutting board. When cool enough to handle, cut into halves.
3. Meanwhile, place a pan over medium heat. Crack the eggs in the pan. Add salt, pepper, and bacon and scramble it. Cook until the eggs are set. Stir frequently.

4. Press the inside of the sweet potato slightly.

5. Place 1 sweet potato half on a microwave-safe plate. Place egg mixture on top.

6. Sprinkle cheese on top. Microwave on high for 30 seconds or until cheese melts.

OAT AND SPELT PUMPKIN MUFFINS

Number of servings: 20

Nutritional values per serving (without optional ingredients):

- Calories: 125
- Fat: 1.5 g
- Carbohydrates: 25 g
- Protein: 4 g

INGREDIENTS:

For wet ingredients:

- 2 flax eggs (2 tablespoons ground flax mixed with 4 table-spoons water)
- ½ cup cashew milk or any other non-dairy milk of your choice
- 2 very large overripe bananas, mashed
- ½ cup pure maple syrup
- 1½ cups pumpkin puree
- 2 teaspoons vanilla extract

FOR DRY INGREDIENTS:

- 2 cups rolled oats or quick oats
- 1 teaspoon baking soda
- 2 teaspoons baking powder
- 2 cups whole-grain spelt flour
- 1 teaspoon baking soda

- 4 teaspoons pumpkin pie spice

OPTIONAL INGREDIENTS:

- 4–6 tablespoons dark chocolate chips, melted
- ¼ cup chopped pecans
- ¼ cup chopped walnuts
- 2 teaspoons chia seeds

DIRECTIONS:

1. Set aside the flax eggs after mixing together flaxseeds and water in the refrigerator for 15 minutes.
2. Remove from the refrigerator and add into a bowl.
3. Add the rest of the wet ingredients and beat with an electric hand mixer until well incorporated and smooth.
4. Add all the dry ingredients into a bowl and stir.
5. Add dry ingredients into the bowl of wet ingredients and beat until just incorporated. Do not overbeat.
6. Grease muffin pans with some ghee or butter.
7. Place disposable liners in it. Pour batter into the muffin pans. Fill them up to ¾ full.
8. Bake in a preheated oven at 375 °F for 20 minutes or until a toothpick comes out clean when inserted in the center.
9. Remove from the oven and place on your countertop for 5 minutes. Place on a cooling rack and cool.
10. Serve warm or at room temperature.
11. Leftovers can be stored in an airtight container in the refrigerator.

RED BERRY AMARANTH PUDDING

Number of servings: 3

Nutritional values per serving:

- Calories: 143.1
- Fat: 1.3 g
- Carbohydrates: 31.5 g
- Protein: 2.8 g

INGREDIENTS:

- ¼ cup amaranth grains, coarsely ground
- 1 piece (1 inch) cinnamon
- 1 tablespoon honey
- Juice of ½ lemon
- A pinch salt
- 1 cup unsweetened apple juice
- 1 cup berries of your choice
- Zest of ½ lemon, grated (optional)

DIRECTIONS:

1. Add amaranth, cinnamon, lemon juice, salt, apple juice, and lemon zest into a saucepan.
2. Place the saucepan over medium-high heat. When it begins to boil, lower heat and cook until slightly thick. Turn off the heat.
3. Discard the cinnamon. Add honey and berries and mix well.
4. Divide into bowls. Cool completely and refrigerate until use.

CHAPTER 9: MEAL RECIPES

PEA AND FARRO STIR-FRY

Number of servings: 2

Nutritional values per serving:

- Calories: 525
- Fat: 20 g
- Carbohydrates: 67 g
- Protein: 27 g

INGREDIENTS:

- 2 cups fresh or frozen peas, thawed
- 1⅓ cups cooked farro
- 4 cloves garlic, minced
- 4 large eggs, beaten
- 4 teaspoons olive oil, divided
- 1 medium sweet onion, thinly sliced
- ½ cup fresh basil, torn
- ½ teaspoon paprika
- Salt and pepper to taste

DIRECTIONS:

1. Place a large cast-iron skillet over medium-high heat. Add 2 teaspoons oil and heat. Crack the eggs and constantly stir until scrambled and cooked.
2. Add garlic, pepper, and salt and sauté until aromatic.
3. Stir in the rest of the ingredients and stir fry for 3–4 minutes.

SPICY CHICKEN AND SPELT SALAD

Number of servings: 5

Nutritional values per serving:

- Calories: 226
- Fat: 10.2 g
- Carbohydrates: 21.8 g
- Protein: 14.2 g

INGREDIENTS:

For dressing:

- 2 tablespoons soy sauce
- 1 tablespoon olive oil
- 1 tablespoon creamy peanut butter
- ½ tablespoon freshly grated ginger
- ½ Serrano chili pepper, minced
- ½ tablespoon grated garlic
- 1½ tablespoons Asian sesame oil
- 1 tablespoon rice wine vinegar
- ¼ teaspoon cayenne pepper

FOR SPELT:

- 3 cups water
- ½ cup spelt kernels
- ¼ teaspoon salt

FOR CHICKEN:

- 2 cups water
- 2 chicken breast halves, skinless, boneless
- ¼ teaspoon salt
- 1 small onion, chopped into chunks

FOR SALAD:

- ½ red bell pepper, sliced
- 2 tablespoons chopped parsley
- 1½ carrots, thinly sliced
- ½ bunch green onions, sliced
- 1 cup thinly sliced red cabbage
- 2 tablespoons chopped parsley

DIRECTIONS:

1. *To make the dressing:* Add all the ingredients for the dressing into a bowl and whisk well.
2. Cover and set aside for a while for the flavors to set in.
3. *To make spelt:* Place a skillet over medium-high heat. Add spelt and stir frequently until brown. A few of them may have popped up.
4. Transfer into a wire mesh strainer. Place the strainer under cold running water and rinse.
5. Add water and salt into a saucepan. Place the saucepan over high heat.

6. When it begins to boil, add spelt. When it again begins to boil, lower heat to low heat and cook until tender.

7. Drain off excess water from the pan. Let it cool completely.

8. Meanwhile, cook the chicken as follows: Pour water into the skillet. Add salt and onion. Place the skillet over medium-high heat.

9. When it begins to boil, add the chicken and lower the heat slightly. Cook until the chicken is done.

10. Remove the chicken with a slotted spoon and then place it on the cutting board. Use the broth in some other recipe.

11. When the chicken is cool enough to handle, shred it with a pair of forks.

12. Place chicken in a large bowl. Add spelt and all the salad ingredients and toss well.

13. Pour dressing on top. Toss well and serve.

LAYERED SPELT SALAD

Number of servings: 4

Nutritional values per serving:

- Calories: 202
- Fat: 11.4 g
- Carbohydrates: 20.5 g
- Protein: 7.8 g

INGREDIENTS:
FOR SALAD:

- 1 cucumber, diced
- 1 cup shredded red cabbage
- 1 cup cooked spelt (follow the previous recipe)
- 1 cup sliced celery
- 1 cup broccoli florets, raw or cooked, as per your preference
- 4 tablespoons sunflower seeds

FOR DRESSING:

- 4 teaspoons olive oil
- ½ teaspoon dried oregano
- ½ teaspoon dried basil
- Freshly ground pepper to taste
- 6 tablespoons plain yogurt
- Salt to taste

DIRECTIONS:

1. *To make the dressing:* Add all the ingredients for the dressing into a bowl and whisk well.

2. Cover and set aside for a while for the flavors to set in.

3. Take 4 mason jars. Layer them with cooked spelt and vegetables in any manner you desire.

4. Divide the dressing into the jars. Scatter sunflower seeds on top. Fasten the lids and refrigerate until use. It can last for 2–3 days.

PIZZA WRAPS

Number of servings: 2

Nutritional values per serving:

- Calories: 146
- Fat: 4 g
- Carbohydrate: 24 g
- Protein: 9 g

INGREDIENTS:

- 2 whole wheat flour tortillas (8 inches each)
- 24 leaves baby spinach
- 4 tablespoons prepared pizza sauce
- 6 tablespoons part-skim mozzarella cheese, shredded

DIRECTIONS:

1. Place tortillas on a large microwave-safe plate or use 2 plates.
2. Divide the pizza sauce among the tortillas. Spread spinach equally on both the tortillas.
3. Divide and sprinkle cheese over the spinach.
4. Microwave on high for 30–40 seconds until cheese melts.
5. Roll the tortillas and place on a plate with its seam side facing down.
6. Serve immediately.

SPICY CHICKEN BREASTS

Number of servings: 2

Nutritional values per serving:

- Calories: 173
- Fat: 2.4 g
- Carbohydrates: 9.2 g
- Protein: 29.2 g

INGREDIENTS:

- 1¼ tablespoons paprika
- ½ tablespoon salt or to taste
- ½ tablespoon dried thyme
- ½ tablespoon ground pepper
- 1 tablespoon garlic powder
- ½ tablespoon onion powder
- ½ tablespoon ground cayenne pepper
- 2 chicken breast halves, skinless and boneless

DIRECTIONS:

1. Add all the spices and salt into a bowl and stir.
2. Sprinkle some of the mixture over the chicken. Rub the spice mixture over the chicken. Use as much as required to suit your taste. The remaining can be stored in an airtight container for future use or use it in some other recipe.

3. Grease a grill grate lightly with oil. Preheat the grill to high heat.

4. Grill the chicken for 6–8 minutes on each side or until the juices are released.

SPICY CAJUN CHICKEN QUINOA

Number of servings: 2

Nutritional values per serving:

- Calories: 386
- Fat: 7 g
- Carbohydrates: 35 g
- Protein: 47 g

INGREDIENTS:

- 2 chicken breasts, cut into bite-size pieces
- ¼ cup quinoa
- ¼ pouch (from a ½-pound pouch) ready-to-use Puy lentils
- 1 red onion, cut into thin wedges
- A handful fresh cilantro, chopped
- ½ tablespoon Cajun seasoning
- 1 ¼ cups hot chicken stock
- ½ tablespoon olive oil
- 1.8 ounces dried apricots, sliced
- ½ bunch spring onions, chopped

DIRECTIONS:

1. Place chicken in a baking dish. Sprinkle Cajun spice over the chicken and toss well.
2. Bake in a preheated oven at 390 °F for 20 minutes or until

cooked.

3. Meanwhile, add quinoa and stock into a saucepan. Place a saucepan over medium heat. Cook until tender.

4. Add apricots and lentils during the last 5 minutes of cooking. Drain excess water and add into a bowl. Add chicken and toss well.

5. Place a pan over medium heat. Add oil and heat. Add onion and sauté until translucent. Transfer into the bowl of quinoa. Add cilantro and spring onions and toss. Serve right away.

CHICKEN WALDORF SALAD

Number of servings: 2

Nutritional values per serving:

- Calories: 762
- Fat: 44 g
- Carbohydrates: 61 g
- Protein: 39 g

INGREDIENTS:

FOR SALAD:

- 1 cup cooked farro
- 1 small apple, cored and diced
- 1 tablespoon dried cherries
- ½ cup almonds, toasted
- ¾ cup diced rotisserie chicken
- 6 tablespoons halved green grapes
- ¾ cup coarsely chopped Bibb lettuce

FOR DRESSING:

- 2 small cloves garlic, peeled, minced
- ¼ teaspoon honey
- ¾ teaspoon Dijon mustard
- ½ tablespoon white wine vinegar
- 3 tablespoons olive oil
- Salt to taste

DIRECTIONS:

1. *To make the dressing:* Add all the ingredients for dressing into a bowl. Whisk well.

2. Cover and set aside for a while so that the flavors set in.

3. Add all the ingredients for the salad, except almonds, into a bowl and toss well.

4. Pour dressing on top and toss well.

5. Divide into plates. Scatter almonds on top and serve.

GREEN GODDESS SOUP

Number of servings: 6

Nutritional values per serving:

- Calories: 169
- Fat: 8.4 g
- Carbohydrates: 17.3 g
- Protein: 10.1 g

INGREDIENTS:

FOR SOUP:

- 12 cups baby spinach or super greens blend
- ½ teaspoon wasabi powder (optional)
- ¼ cup peeled, sliced fresh ginger
- ½ teaspoon turmeric powder
- ½ teaspoon cayenne pepper
- 2 cloves garlic, peeled
- 2 cups chicken broth or vegetable broth
- 1 cup coconut milk
- 2–3 teaspoons lemon or lime juice
- Salt and pepper to taste

FOR GARNISH:

- 2 cups broccoli florets, lightly steamed
- ½ cup Greek yogurt, diluted with milk
- Chia seeds

DIRECTIONS:

1. Add all the ingredients into a blender and blend until smooth and well combined.
2. Pour into a saucepan. Place the saucepan over medium heat. Heat thoroughly. Stir frequently.
3. Taste and adjust the seasoning and lemon juice if necessary.
4. Ladle into soup bowls. Scatter broccoli florets in each bowl. Drizzle some yogurt and sprinkle chia seeds. Swirl lightly.
5. Serve.

GRILLED LAMB SKEWERS WITH WARM FAVA BEAN SALAD

Number of servings: 3

Nutritional values per serving (2 skewers with ½-cup salad and a lemon wedge):

- Calories: 284
- Fat: 10.3 g
- Carbohydrate: 23 g
- Protein: 24.8 g

INGREDIENTS:

- ¾ pound leg of lamb, cut into 1-inch cubes
- 2 cups shelled fava beans (about 2 pounds unshelled)
- A handful of fresh mint leaves, chopped
- 1 tablespoon fresh lemon juice
- ½ teaspoon lemon rind, grated
- ¾ teaspoon extra-virgin olive oil
- ½ teaspoon salt, divided
- 1 tablespoon water
- 3 lemon wedges
- ¼ teaspoon freshly ground pepper, divided
- Low-calorie cooking spray

DIRECTIONS:

1. Place a pot half-filled with water over high heat. When it begins to boil, add fava beans and cook for a minute or until it is tender. Drain and place under cold running water for a couple of minutes. Drain again.

2. Discard the outer skin from the beans.

3. *To make the dressing:* Add oil, lemon juice, lemon rind, mint, ¼ teaspoon salt and, ⅛ teaspoon pepper into a small bowl and whisk well.

4. Place a saucepan over medium-high heat. Add beans and tablespoon water and cook for a couple of minutes.

5. Transfer into a bowl. Pour dressing on top and toss well.

6. Meanwhile, set up a grill and let it preheat. Grease the grill grates with cooking spray.

7. Spray lamb pieces with cooking spray. Season with remaining salt and pepper.

8. Thread the lamb onto the skewers. Place the skewers on the grill. Grill for 7–8 minutes or until cooked through. Turn the skewers occasionally.

9. Serve lamb with warm fava salad and lemon wedges.

FISH TACOS

Number of servings: 2

Nutritional values per serving:

- Calories: 363
- Fat: 12 g
- Carbohydrates: 28 g
- Protein: 38 g

INGREDIENTS:

- ½ tablespoon olive oil, plus extra for grilling
- ½ teaspoon ground coriander
- 3 radishes, sliced
- 2 tilapia or halibut or black bass fillets (6 ounces each)
- 1 small cucumber, cut into half-moons
- 4 corn tortillas, warmed
- 2 tablespoons sour cream
- 1 tablespoon fresh lime juice
- Lime wedges to serve
- ½ cup chopped cilantro leaves
- Kosher salt and pepper to taste

DIRECTIONS:

1. Preheat a grill to high heat. Grease the grill grates with some oil.
2. Sprinkle salt, pepper, and coriander over the fillets and place

on the preheated grill.

3. Cook for 1–2 minutes on each side.

4. Remove fish from the grill and place on your cutting board. When cool enough to handle, cut into pieces.

5. Meanwhile, make cucumber relish by adding radish, cucumber, oil, salt, pepper, and lime juice into a bowl and toss well.

6. Divide the fish among the tortillas. Sprinkle cilantro. Drizzle sour cream on top.

7. Serve with cucumber relish and lime wedges.

BLACK BEAN, AMARANTH, AVOCADO, MANGO SALAD TOSTADA

Number of servings: 4

Nutritional values per serving:

- Calories: 208.8
- Fat: 5.2 g
- Carbohydrates: 34.2 g
- Protein: 6.1 g

INGREDIENTS:

- ½ can (from a 15-ounce can) black beans, drained and rinsed
- 1 cup water
- ½ cup dry amaranth seeds
- ½ Mexican avocado, peeled, pitted, chopped
- ½ jalapeño pepper, sliced
- 2 small plum tomatoes, chopped
- Juice of a lime
- A handful cilantro, chopped
- 4 corn tortillas, to serve
- Salt and pepper to taste

DIRECTIONS:

1. Add water and amaranth seeds into a saucepan. Place the saucepan over medium heat. Cook until dry. Turn off the heat.

2. Add into a bowl. Add the rest of the ingredients and toss well.

3. Spread tortillas on your countertop. Top with amaranth mixture and serve.

EDAMAME, AMARANTH, AND CHIMICHURRI NOURISH BOWL

Number of servings: 2

Nutritional values per serving:

- Calories: 370
- Fat: 11.1 g
- Carbohydrates: 54.2 g
- Protein: 19.4 g

INGREDIENTS:

FOR CHIMICHURRI DRESSING:

- ½ bunch cilantro, chopped
- 2 small cloves garlic, peeled
- Juice of ½ lemon
- ½ tablespoon olive oil
- Salt to taste

FOR AMARANTH:

- 1¼ cups water
- ½ cup amaranth
- ½ tablespoon loose vegetable bouillon

FOR VEGETABLES:

- ½ zucchini, cut into round slices
- ½ red onion, thinly sliced

- ½ small head cauliflower, cut into florets
- ½ red bell pepper, cut into 1-inch squares
- 1 cup edamame
- 1 small carrot, grated
- ½ bunch spinach
- Cooking spray

DIRECTIONS:

1. *To cook amaranth:* Add amaranth and water into a pot. Place the pot over medium heat.
2. When it begins to boil, add amaranth and cook until dry.
3. Meanwhile, add all the ingredients for dressing into a blender and blend until smooth and thick.
4. Add zucchini, bell pepper, onion, and cauliflower into a bowl and toss well. Pour half the chimichurri dressing over the vegetables and toss lightly.
5. Grease a roasting pan with cooking spray. Spread the vegetables in the pan. Spread it evenly.
6. Bake in a preheated oven at 400 °F for 20 minutes.
7. Transfer into a mixing bowl. Add amaranth, edamame, carrot, and spinach and toss well.
8. Pour remaining dressing on top. Fold gently and serve.

STIR-FRIED THAI TOFU SORGHUM BOWL

Number of servings: 2

Nutritional values per serving:

- Calories: 416
- Fat: 16 g
- Carbohydrates: 54 g
- Protein: 20 g

INGREDIENTS:

FOR SORGHUM BOWL:

- 2 teaspoons peanut oil, divided
- 1 carrot, peeled and sliced
- 1 clove garlic, minced
- ½ red bell pepper, sliced
- 1 cup chopped asparagus spears
- ½ tablespoon grated ginger
- ½ tablespoon water
- ¾ cup sliced snow peas
- ½ package (from a 15-ounce package) extra-firm tofu, pressed of excess moisture, cut into 1-inch cubes
- ½ tablespoon soy sauce
- 1 cup cooked sorghum, cooked according to the instructions on the package

FOR THAI SAUCE:

- ½ cup light canned coconut milk
- 3 tablespoons creamy peanut butter
- 1¼ tablespoons pure maple syrup
- ½ teaspoon cornstarch
- ½ tablespoon Thai red curry paste
- ½ tablespoon soy sauce
- 1 teaspoon minced fresh ginger
- 2 small cloves garlic, peeled and minced

DIRECTIONS:

1. *For sorghum bowl:* Place a nonstick skillet over medium-high heat. Add 1 teaspoon peanut oil and heat. Stir in carrots, asparagus, ginger, and garlic and cook for a minute, stirring constantly.

2. Pour water and stir. Cover and cook for a couple of minutes. Stir in the snow peas, red pepper, and soy sauce. Stir-fry for 3–4 minutes until the vegetables are crisp as well as tender. Transfer into a bowl.

3. Clean the skillet and place it back over medium heat.

4. Pour remaining oil and heat. Swirl the pan so that the oil spreads. Add tofu and cook until light brown and crisp all over. Stir occasionally.

5. *To make Thai sauce:* Add all the ingredients for Thai sauce into a bowl and whisk well.

6. Transfer the sauce into the skillet. Mix well. Add the cooked vegetables and mix well. Heat thoroughly. Turn off the heat.

7. *To assemble:* Place equal amounts of sorghum into 2 serving bowls.

8. Divide the vegetable and tofu mixture among the bowls.

9. Serve hot.

BEEFY CORN AND BLACK BEAN CHILI

Number of servings: 3

Nutritional values per serving:

- Calories: 193
- Fat: 3 g
- Carbohydrates: 20 g
- Protein: 20 g

INGREDIENTS:

- ½ pound ground beef
- ½ package (from a 14-ounce package) frozen seasoned corn
- ½ can (from a 15-ounce can) black beans, drained and rinsed
- ½ can (from a 15-ounce can) seasoned tomato sauce
- 1 green onion, sliced, to serve (optional)
- 1 teaspoon chili powder
- ½ can (from a 14-ounce can) fat-free beef broth
- Low-fat sour cream to garnish (optional)

DIRECTIONS:

1. Place a soup pot over medium-high heat. Add beef and chili powder. Blend and cook until brown. Break it simultaneously as it cooks. Discard the fat remaining in the pot.
2. Add rest of the ingredients and stir. When it begins to boil, lower the heat and cover with a lid. Simmer until thick. Stir

occasionally.

3. Serve in bowls. Garnish with green onion and sour cream if using and serve.

ROAST PORK WITH APPLES AND ONIONS

Number of servings: 4

Nutritional values per serving:

- Calories: 210
- Fat: 7 g
- Carbohydrates: 14 g
- Protein: 23 g

INGREDIENTS:

- 1 pound pork loin roast
- ½ tablespoon olive oil
- 1 large onion, cut into wedges of ¾ inch thick
- ½ tablespoon fresh minced rosemary or ½ teaspoon dried rosemary, crushed
- 1½ large golden delicious apples, cored and cut into 1-inch wedges
- 3 cloves garlic, peeled
- Salt and pepper to taste

DIRECTIONS:

1. Season the roast with salt and pepper.
2. Place an ovenproof skillet over medium heat. Add oil and heat. Add pork and cook until brown all over. Turn off the heat.
3. Scatter apples, garlic, and onions all around the roast. Scatter

rosemary all over.

4. Roast in a preheated oven at 350 °F until the internal temperature shows 145 °F (about 30 minutes). Turn the apple, garlic, and onion halfway through roasting.

5. Remove the skillet from the oven and cover loosely with foil. Let it rest for 10 minutes.

6. Slice the roast and serve with apple, garlic, and onion mixture.

JALAPENO POPPER-CHICKEN PANINI

Number of servings: 2

Nutritional values per serving:

- Calories: 407
- Fat: 18 g
- Carbohydrates: 27 g
- Protein: 33 g

INGREDIENTS:

- 1 skinless, boneless chicken breast (8 ounces), trimmed, halved crosswise
- 1 tablespoon canola oil or avocado oil, divided
- ¼ cup finely chopped pickled jalapeños
- 1 medium tomato, cut into 4 round slices
- ¼ cup low fat whipped cream cheese
- 4 slices crusty whole wheat bread
- Salt and pepper to taste

DIRECTIONS:

1. Place a plastic wrap on your countertop. Place chicken on it. Place another plastic wrap over the chicken and pound it with a meat mallet (from the smooth side) until ¼ inch in thickness.
2. Season chicken with salt and pepper.
3. Place a skillet over medium-high heat. Add half the oil and

heat. Place chicken in the skillet and cook for 3–4 minutes. Flip to the other side and cook for 3–4 minutes. Remove onto a plate. Set aside.

4. Add cream cheese and jalapeño in a bowl and mix well.

5. Divide the mixture equally and spread on each bread slice. Place a chicken each on 2 bread slices. Place 2 tomato slices over each of the chicken.

6. Cover with the remaining bread slices, with the cream cheese side facing down.

7. Brush the remaining oil on both sides of the sandwiches.

8. Place in a preheated panini maker. Cook for 2–3 minutes depending on the desired doneness.

SPINACH-ARTICHOKE-SAUSAGE CAULIFLOWER GNOCCHI

Number of servings: 2

Nutritional values per serving:

- Calories: 261
- Fat: 12 g
- Carbohydrates: 24 g
- Protein: 14 g

INGREDIENTS:

- ½ package (from a 10-ounce package) frozen chopped spinach, thawed and squeezed of excess moisture
- ½ package (from a 12-ounce package) frozen cauliflower gnocchi
- ½ can (from a 14-ounce can) artichoke hearts, drained, quartered
- ½ tablespoon olive oil
- 1 link cooked Italian turkey sausage, drained
- 2 tablespoons freshly grated Parmesan cheese

DIRECTIONS:

1. Place a skillet over medium-high heat. Add oil and heat. Stir in gnocchi and cook until brown. Stir often.
2. Add sausage, spinach, and artichoke hearts and mix well. Cook until spinach wilts.
3. Garnish with Parmesan and serve.

SLOPPY TACOS

Number of servings: 3

Nutritional values per serving: 2 tacos without optional toppings

- Calories: 264
- Fat: 10 g
- Carbohydrates: 17 g
- Protein: 25 g

INGREDIENTS:

- ¾-pound extra-lean ground beef
- ½ teaspoon garlic powder
- Cayenne pepper to taste
- ½ can (from a 15-ounce can) tomato sauce
- 6 taco shells, warmed, to serve
- Salt and pepper to taste

OPTIONAL TOPPINGS:

- Chopped avocado
- Chopped tomatoes
- Shredded cheese
- Salsa
- Shredded lettuce
- Any other toppings of your choice

DIRECTIONS:

1. Place a skillet over medium heat. Cook until it is not pink anymore.
2. Add the rest of the ingredients except taco shells and mix well.
3. When it begins to boil, lower heat and cook for 5–6 minutes.
4. Place ¼-cup meat mixture in each of the tacos. Place optional toppings if desired and serve.

CONCLUSION

O n that note, we have come to the end of this book. I want to thank you once again for choosing this book. I hope it proved to be an enjoyable and informative read and you got all the information you needed about intermittent fasting for women.

In this book, you were given all the information you need about intermittent fasting. Once you understand the way intermittent fasting works, it becomes easier to understand your body's metabolism. This diet works along with your metabolism to improve your overall health. Select a method of fasting that meets your needs and requirements. You don't have to make any drastic changes; you merely need to be mindful of when you eat. If you eat healthy and wholesome meals during the eating window, you will see an improvement in your overall health in no time.

All the recipes given in this book are easy to follow and will help cook tasty and nutritious meals. Now, all that's left is to ensure that you stock up your pantry with the necessary ingredients for cooking delicious meals. By following intermittent fasting, you can eat your way to good health and weight loss! So why don't you get started today?

Thank you and all the best!

REFERENCES

Bjornsdottir, A. (2019). The beginner's guide to the 5:2 diet. Retrieved from https://www.healthline.com/nutrition/the-5-2-diet-guide

Fleck, A. (2019). The disadvantages of fasting. Retrieved from https://healthyeating.sfgate.com/disadvantages-fasting-5546.html

Fung, J., & Eenfeldt, A. (2019). Intermittent fasting for beginners: The complete guide. Retrieved from https://www.dietdoctor.com/intermittent-fasting

Gunnars, K. (2019). 10 evidence-based health benefits of intermittent fasting. Retrieved from https://www.healthline.com/nutrition/10-health-benefits-of-intermittent-fasting

Gustin, A. (2019). 16/8 intermittent fasting: How to do it & get the health benefits. Retrieved from https://perfectketo.com/16-8-intermittent-fasting-ketosis/

How to break a fast safely: Step-by-step guide to breaking a fast (2019). Retrieved from http://siimland.com/how-to-break-a-fast-safely/

How to fast safely: Considerations before starting a fast (2019). Retrieved from https://www.globalhealingcenter.com/natural-health/how-to-fast-safely-considerations-before-fasting/

Mychal, A. (2019). 9 common intermittent fasting mistakes. Retrieved from https://anthonymychal.com/intermittent-fasting-mistakes/

Olsen, N. (2019). One meal a day: Health benefits and risks. Retrieved from https://www.medicalnewstoday.com/articles/320125.php

Oshin, M. (2019). 11 lessons I've learned from 4 years of intermittent fasting: The good and bad. Retrieved from https://mayooshin.com/intermittent-fasting-lessons-learned/

Romaniello, J. (2019). Intermittent fasting FAQ: Top 5 questions about IF Answered. Retrieved from http://romanfitnesssystems.com/articles/intermittent-fasting-faq/

What can you drink while fasting without breaking the fast (2019). Retrieved from http://siimland.com/what-can-you-drink-while-fasting/

What foods are best to eat on an intermittent fasting diet?. (2019). Retrieved from https://greatist.com/eat/what-to-eat-on-an-intermittent-fasting-diet#3

Whittel, N. (2019). The 12 important benefits of autophagy. Retrieved from https://www.naomiwhittel.com/the-12-important-benefits-of-autophagy/

Made in the USA
Middletown, DE
30 December 2019